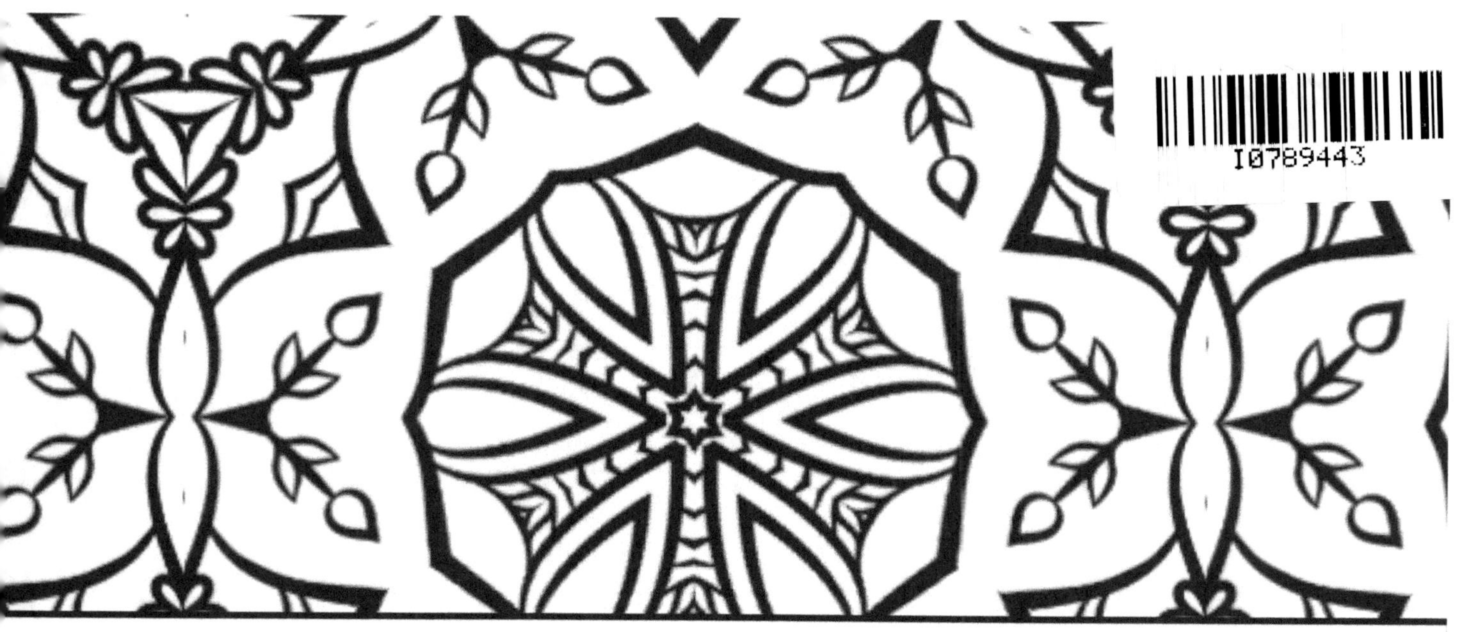

Geriatric Mental Health

Coloring Book For Adults

Volume 1

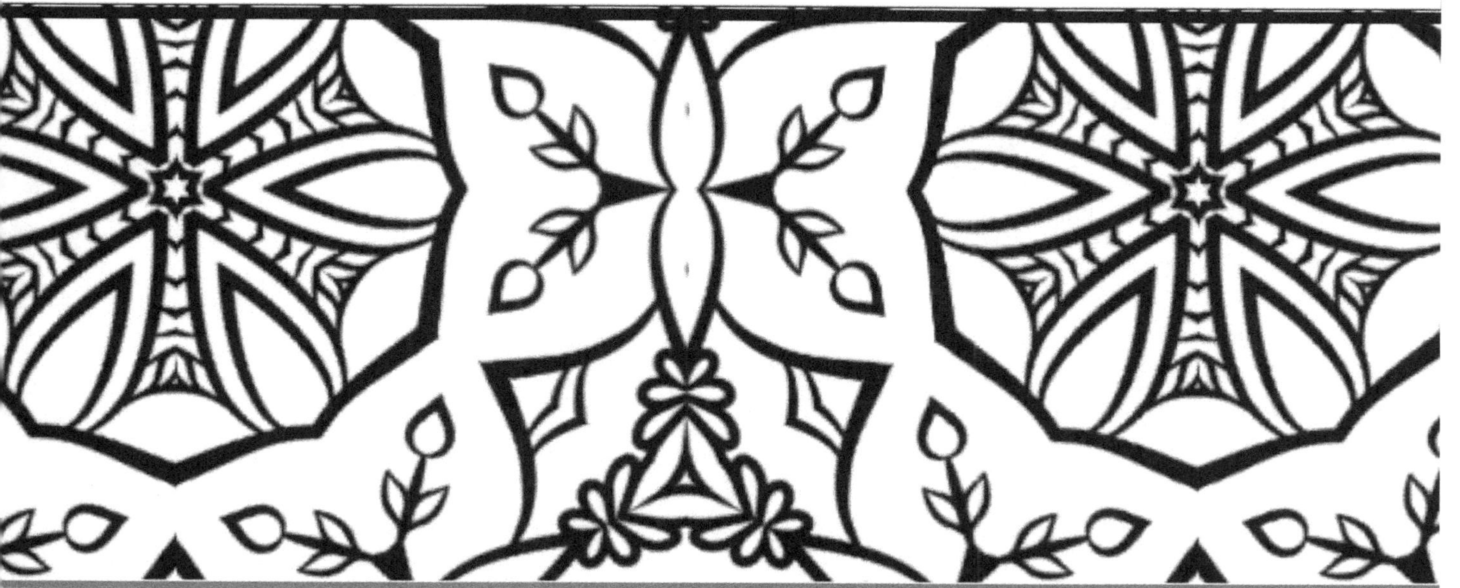

Elizabeth M. Forbes

- Geriatric and Adult Mental Health Professional -

Geriatric Mental Health Coloring Book For Adults – Volume 1
ISBN 13 – 978-1-943833-12-2
ISBN 10 - 1-943833-12-5
Copyright 2017 © by Elizabeth M. Forbes

Published by:
KPLA Publishing – Kissed Publications
PO Box 9819
Hampton, VA 23670
www.kplapublishing.com

10 9 8 7 6 5 4 3 2 1

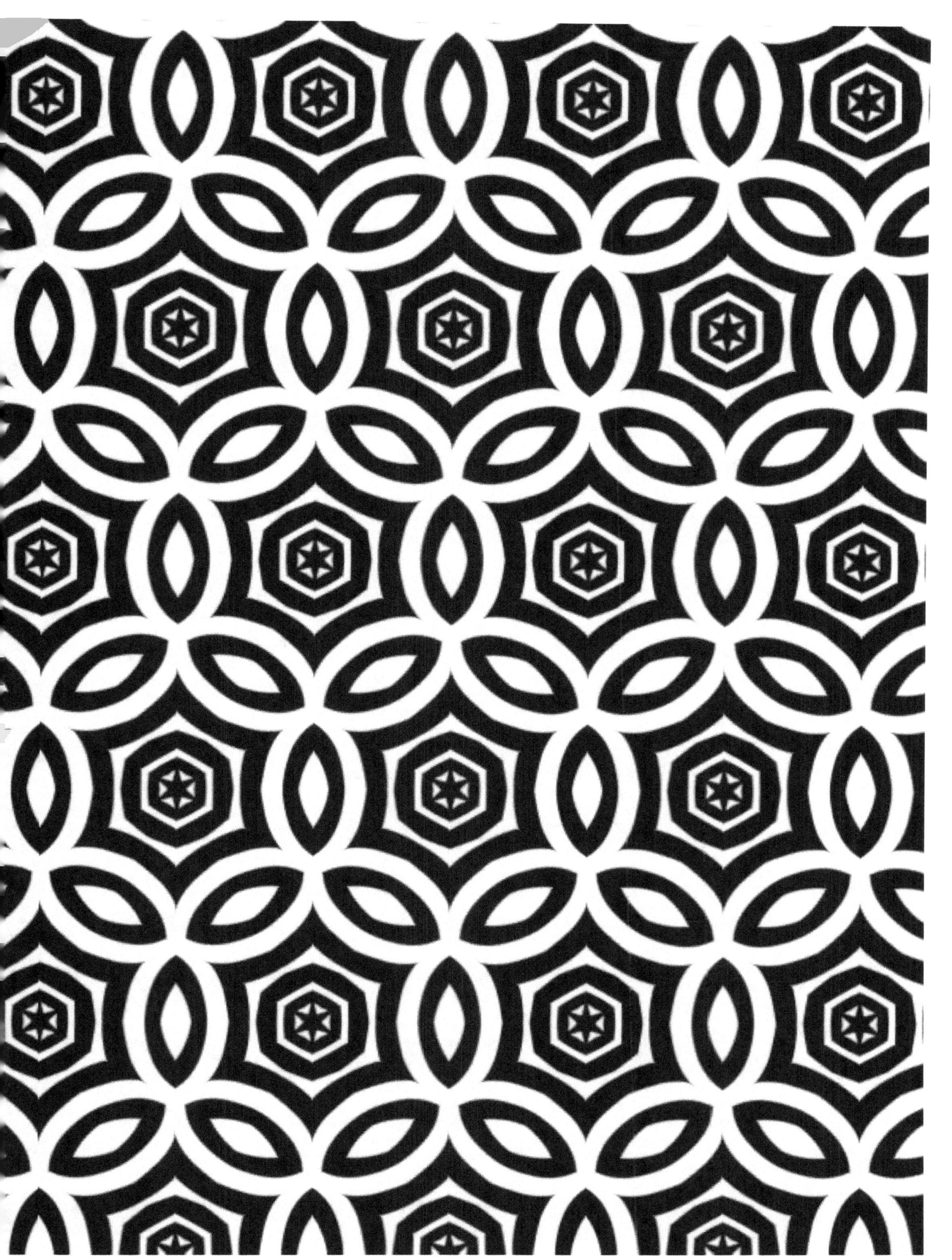

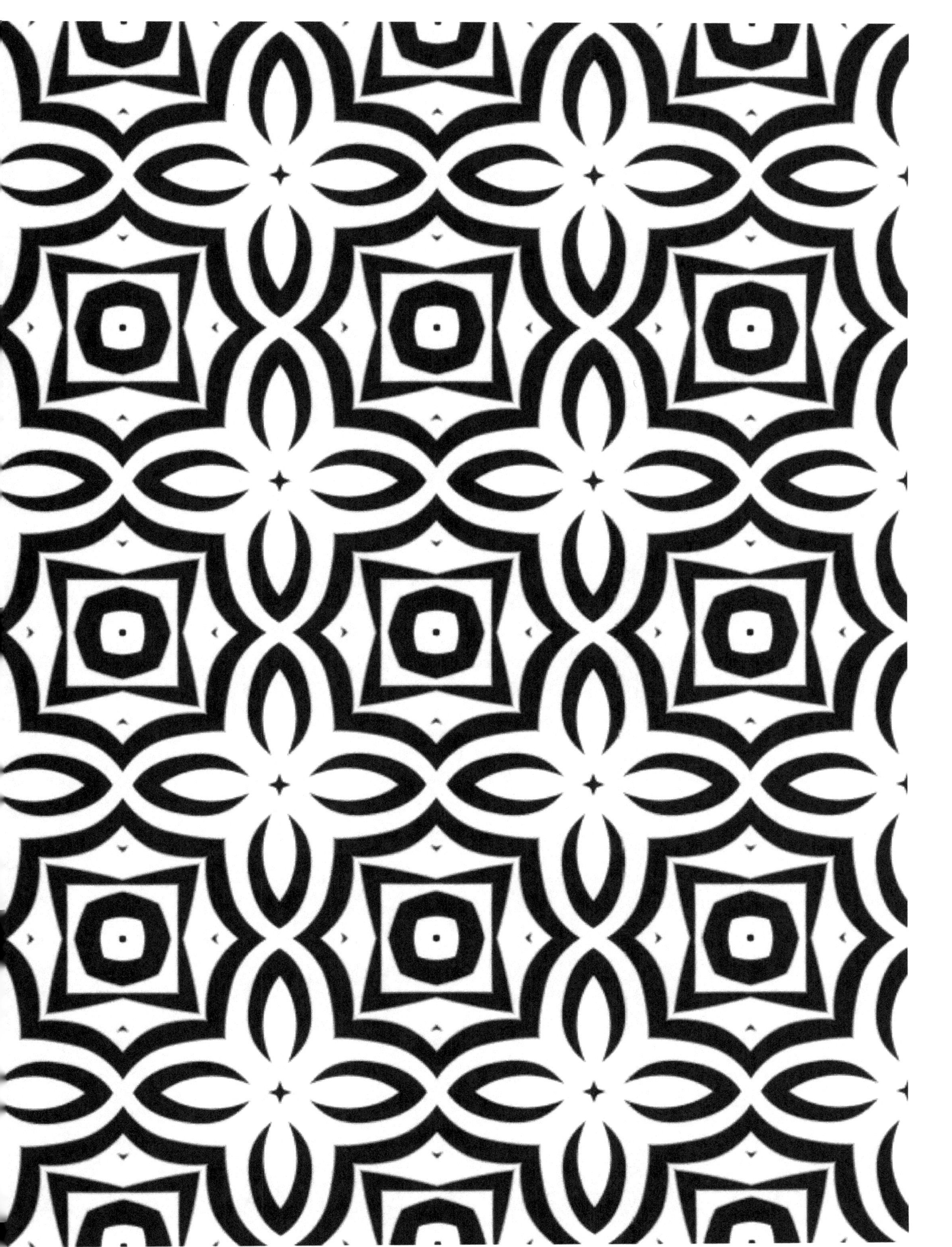

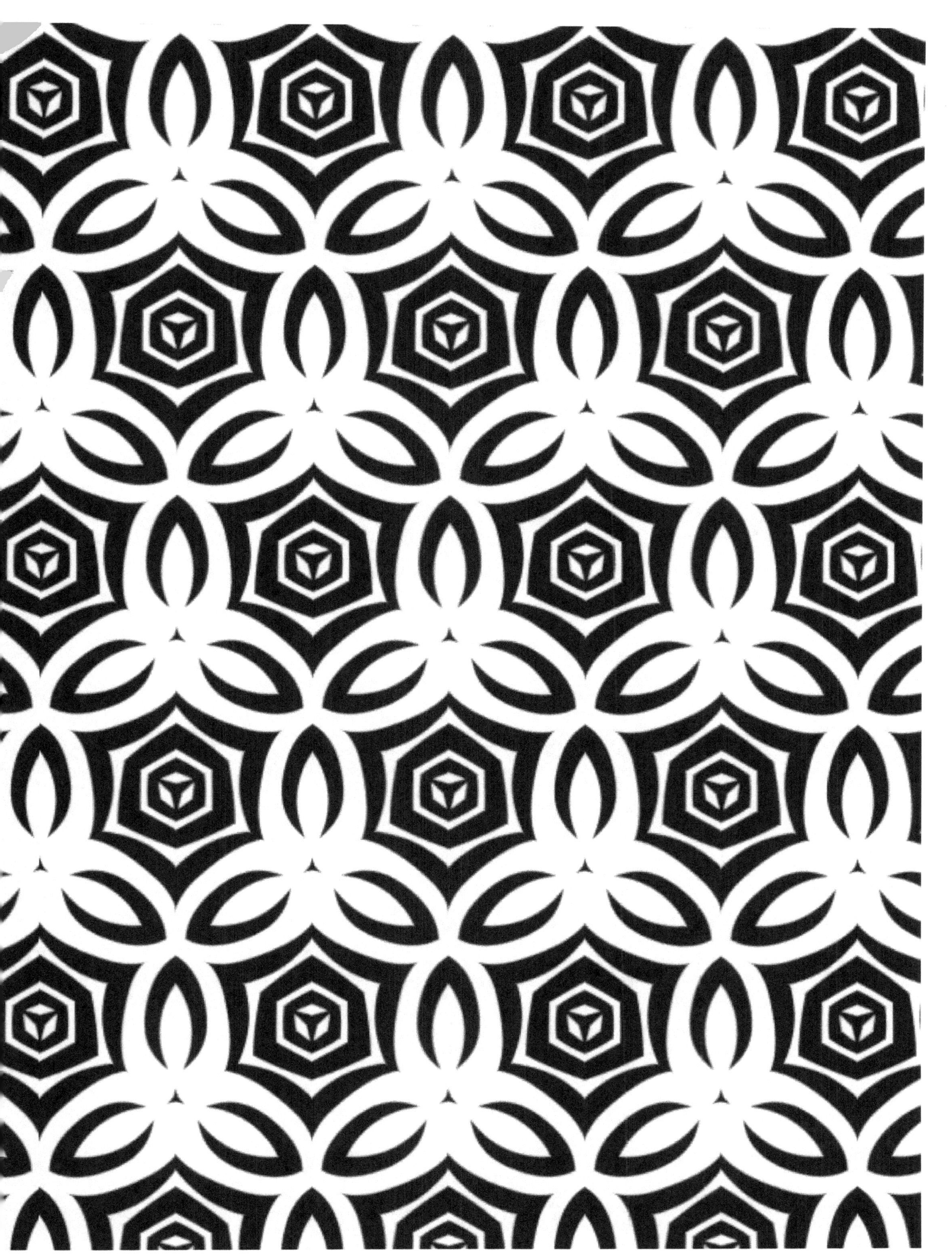

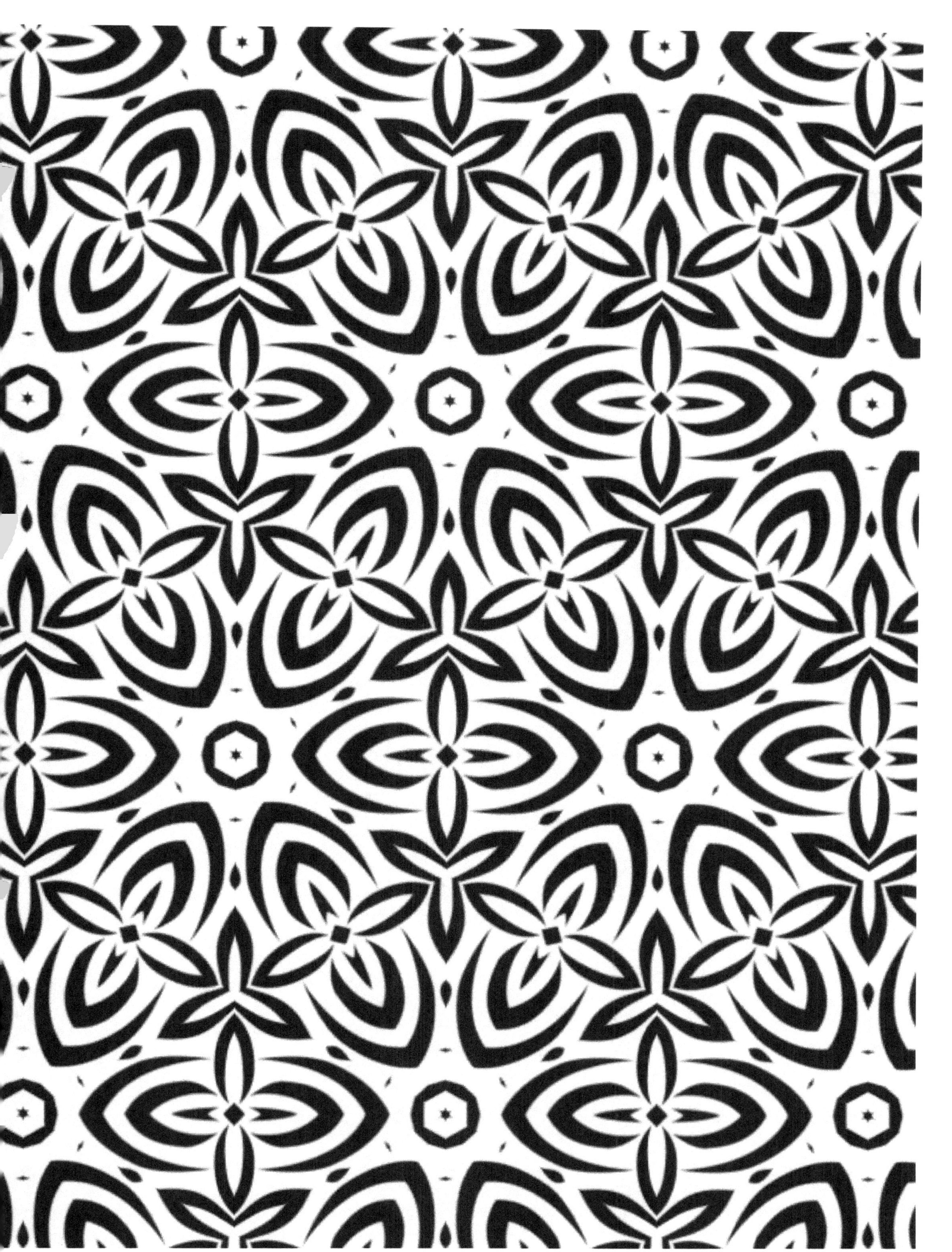

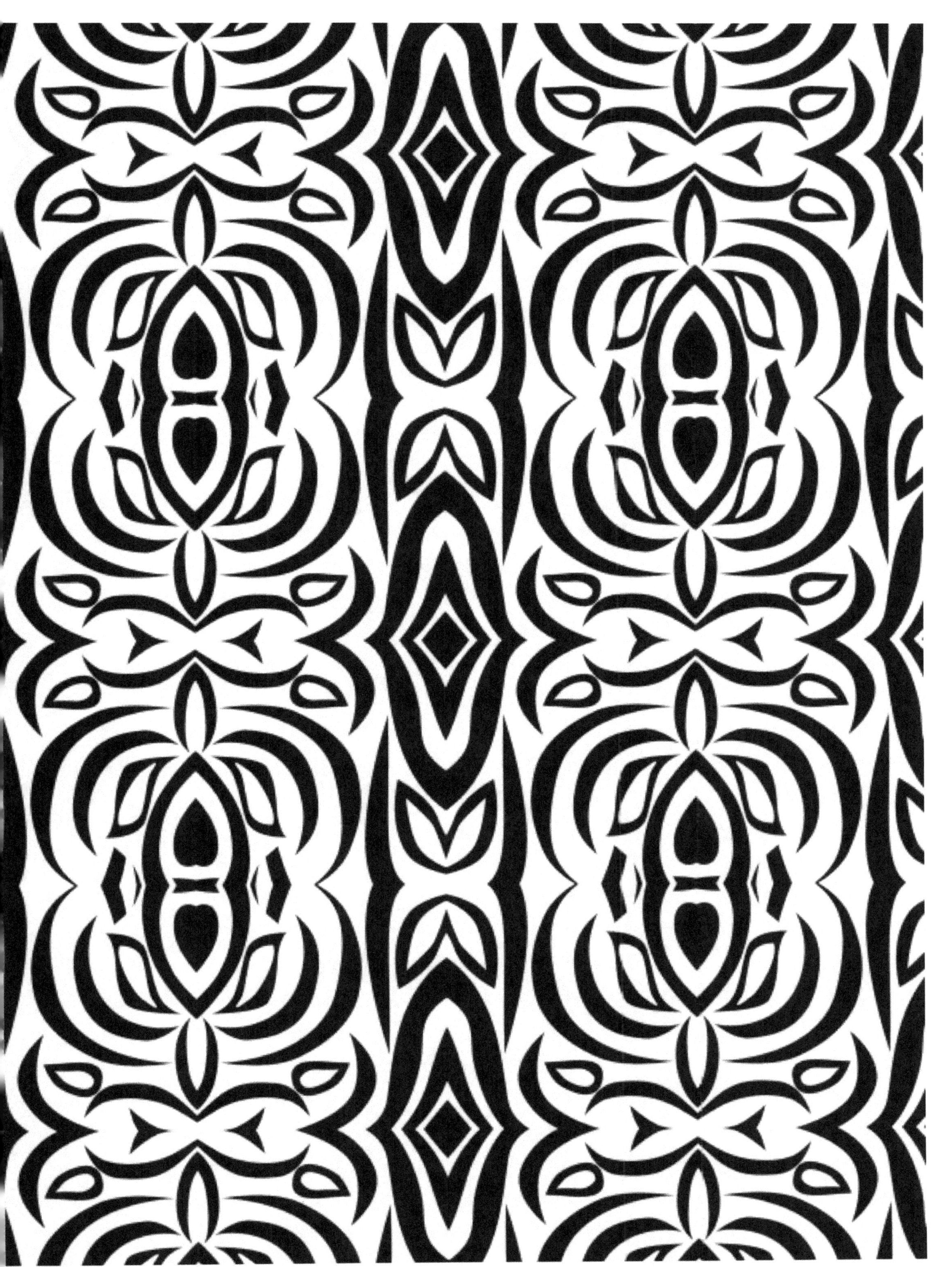

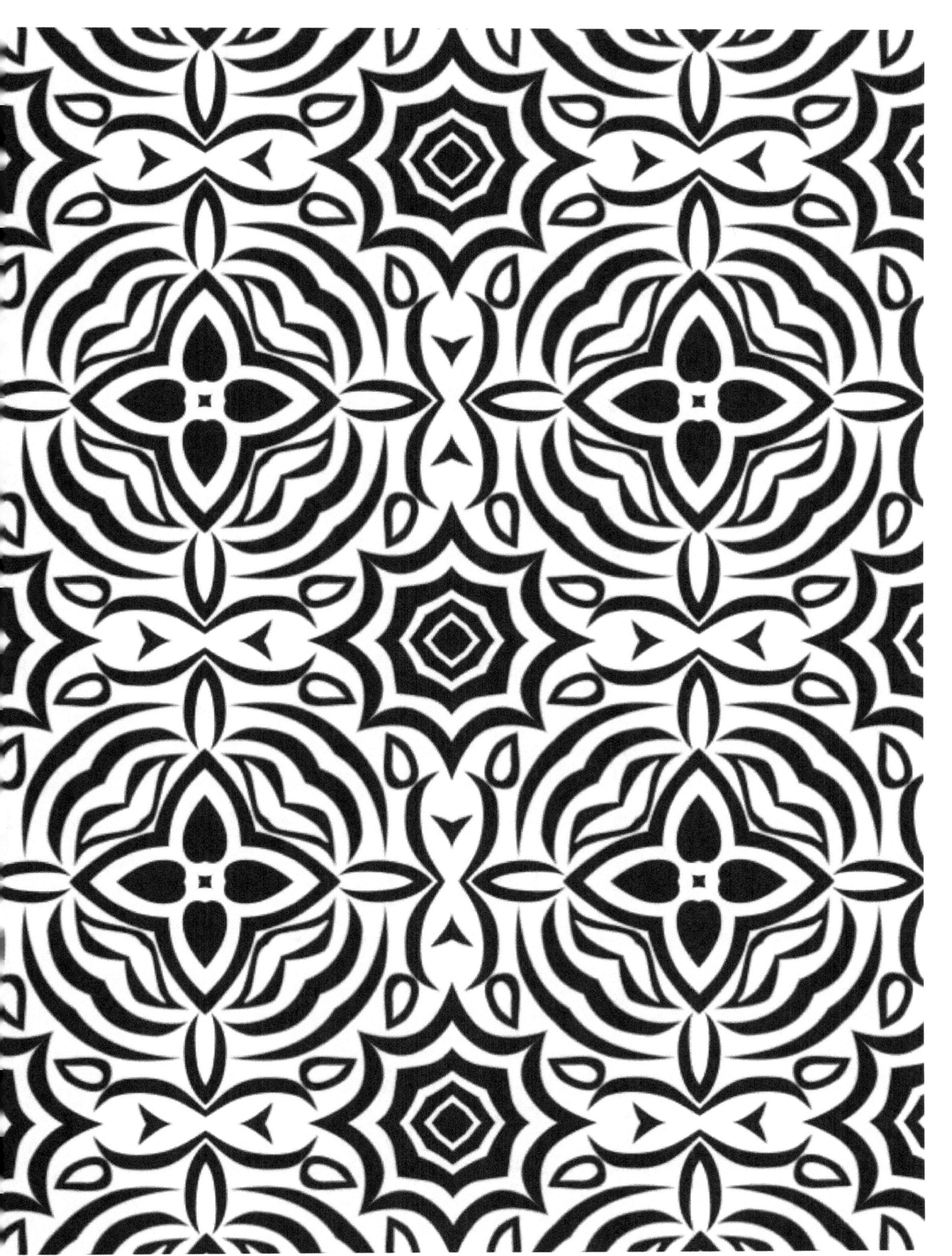

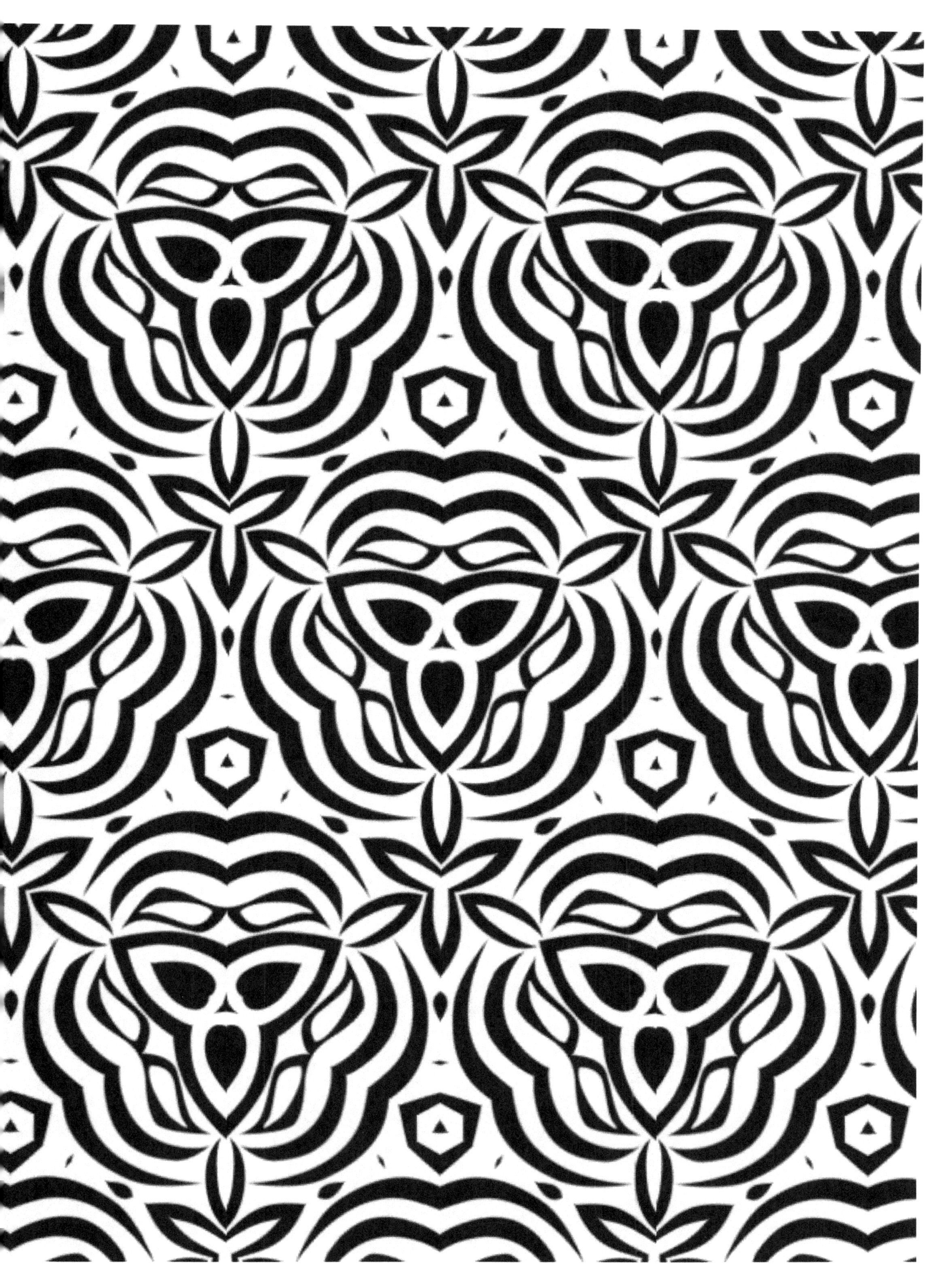

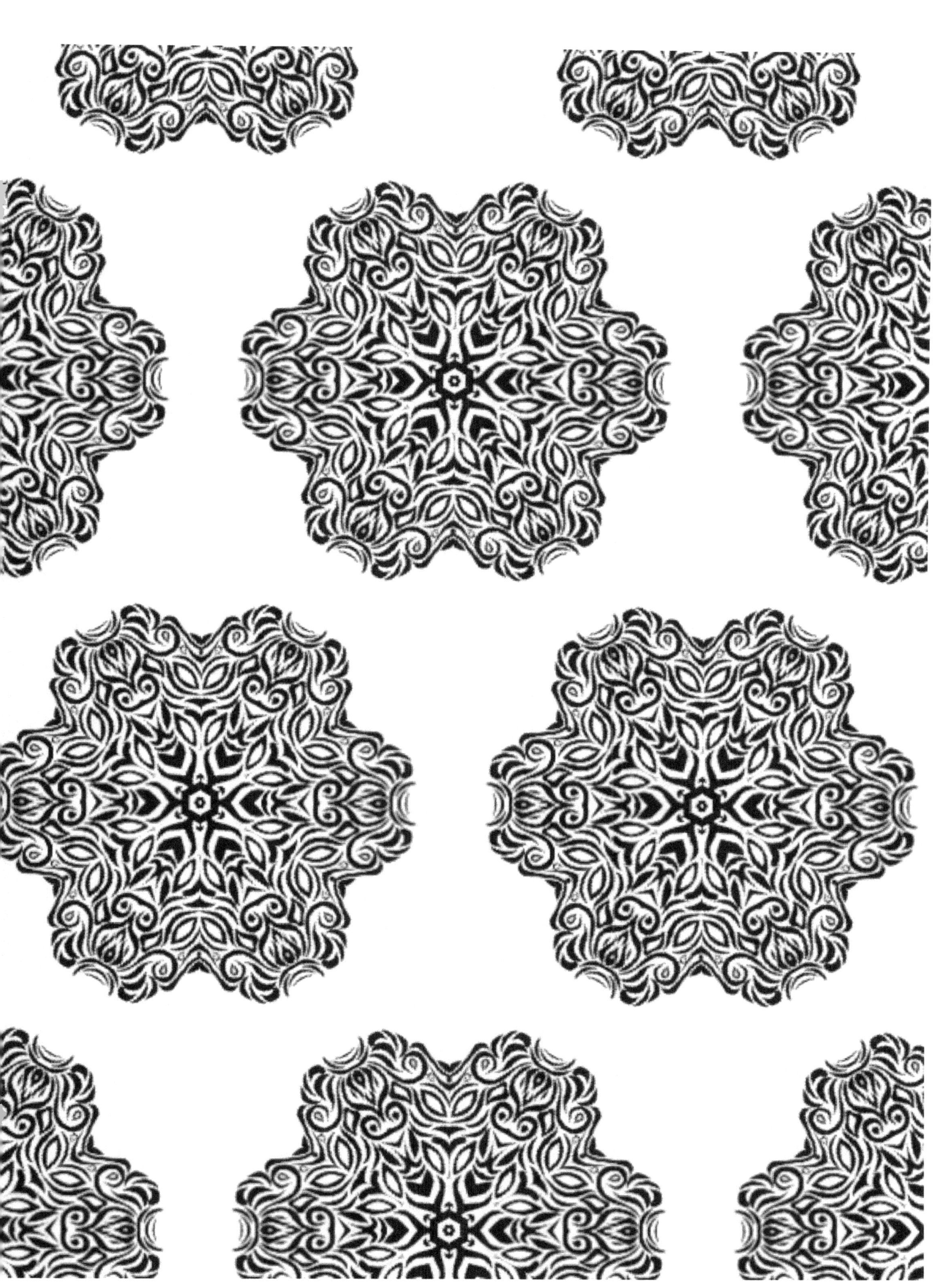

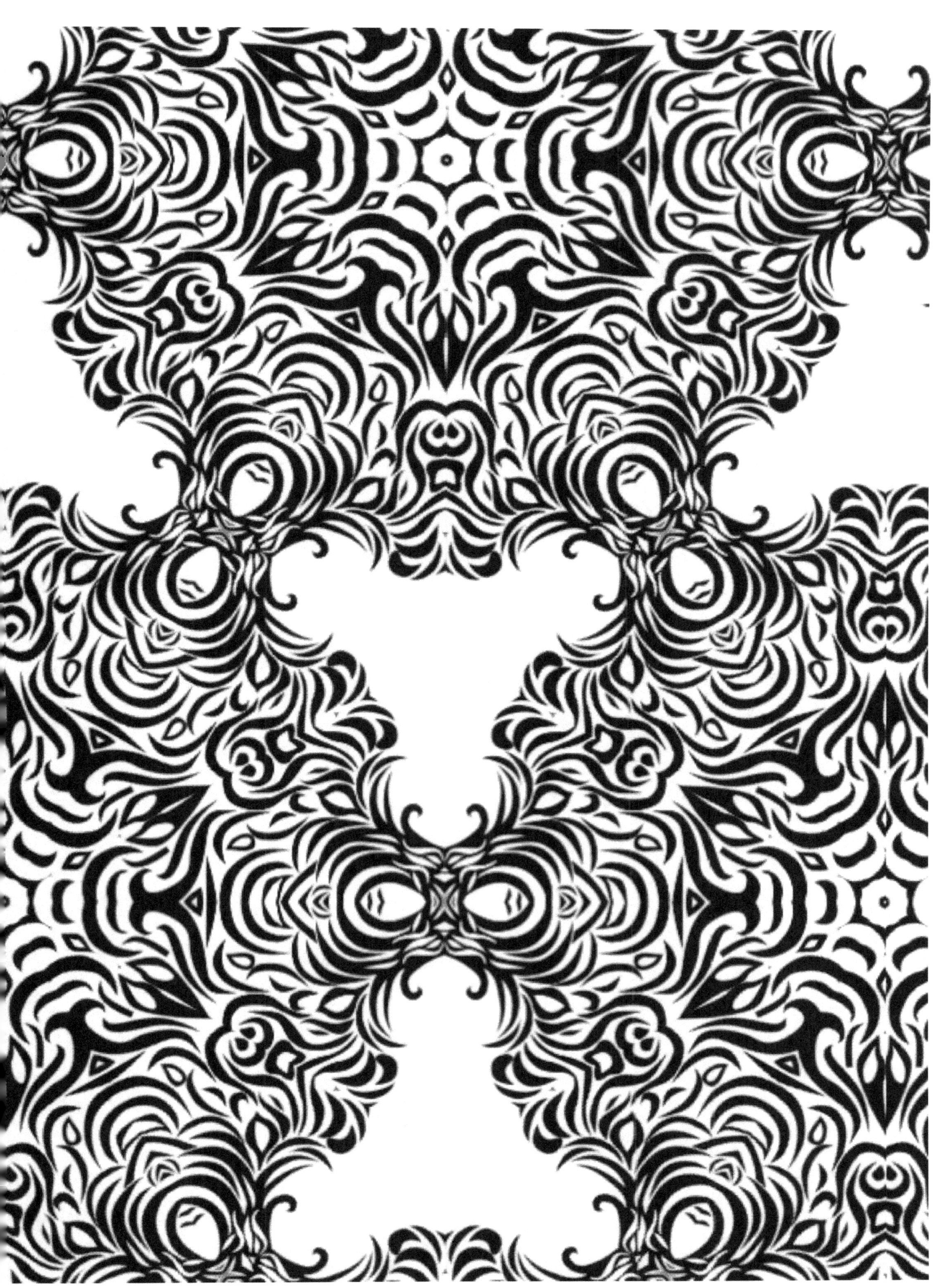

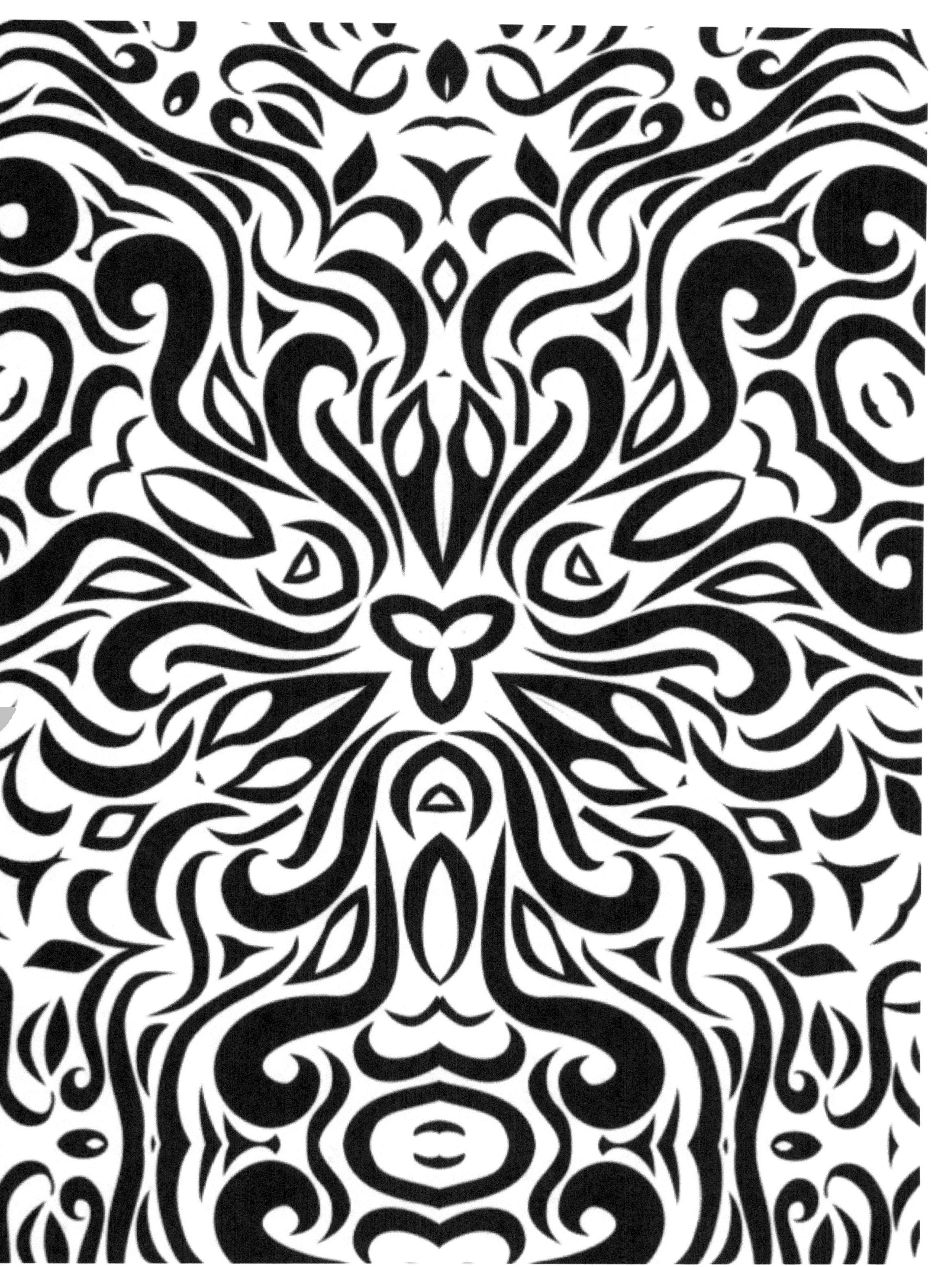

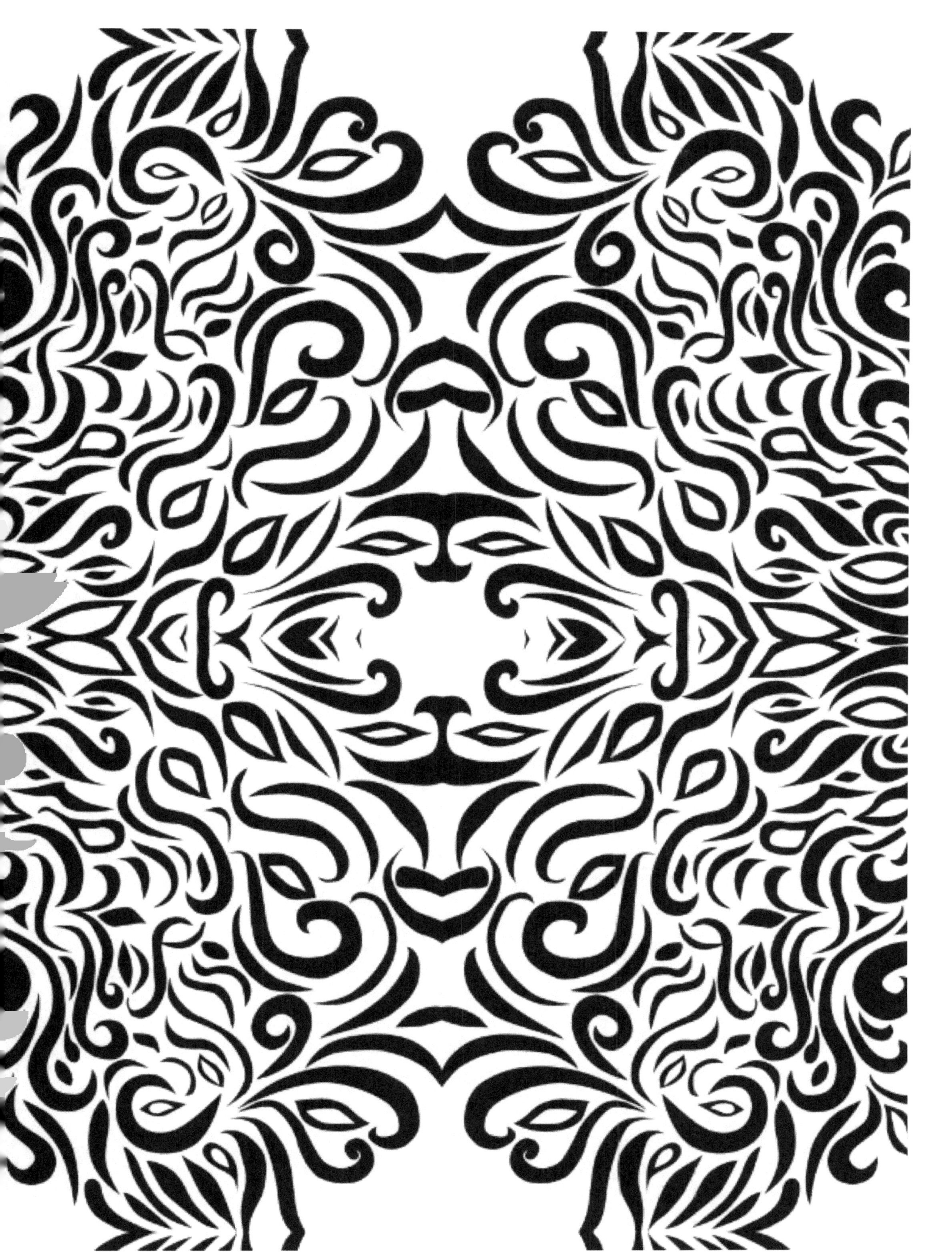

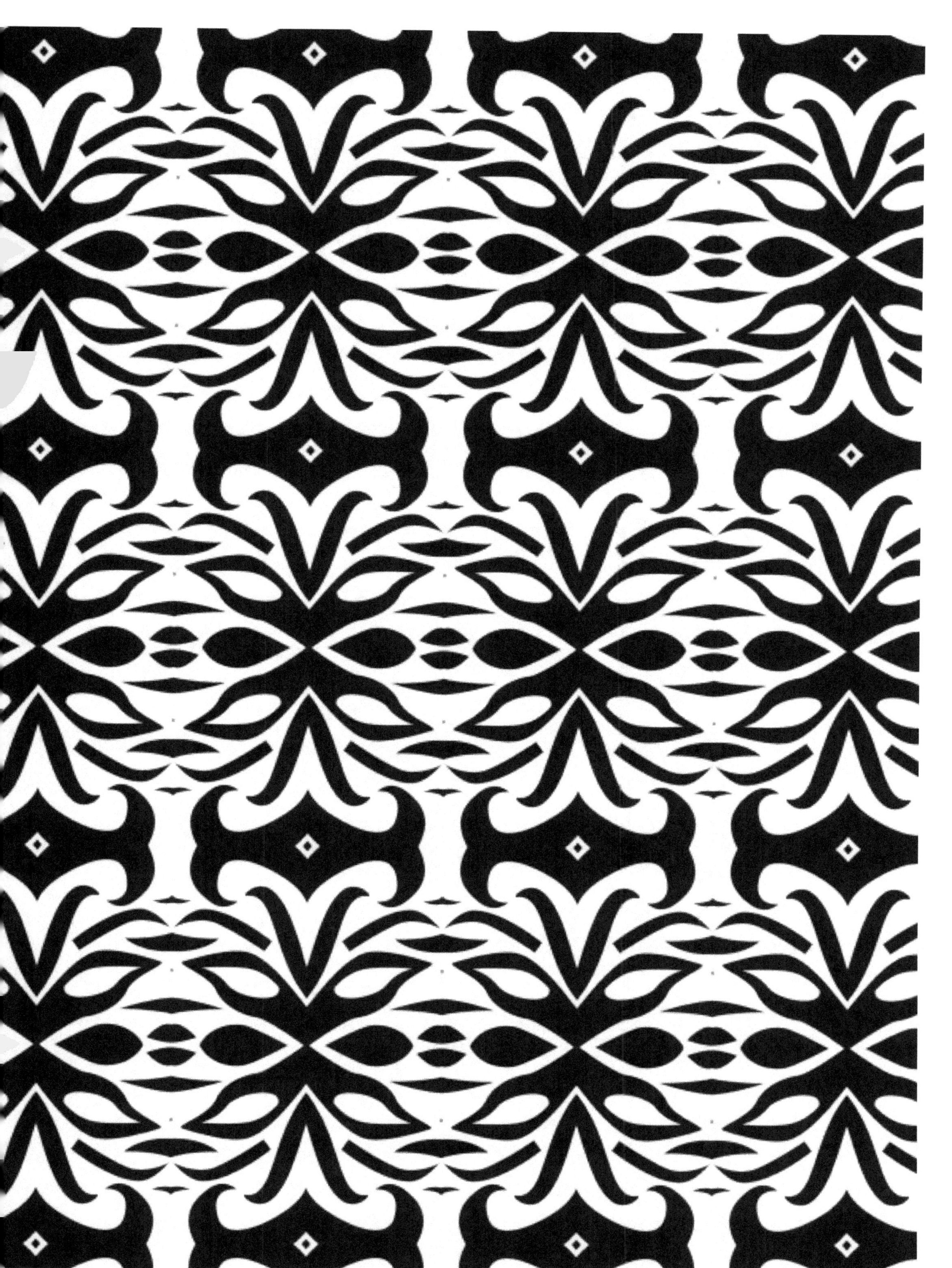

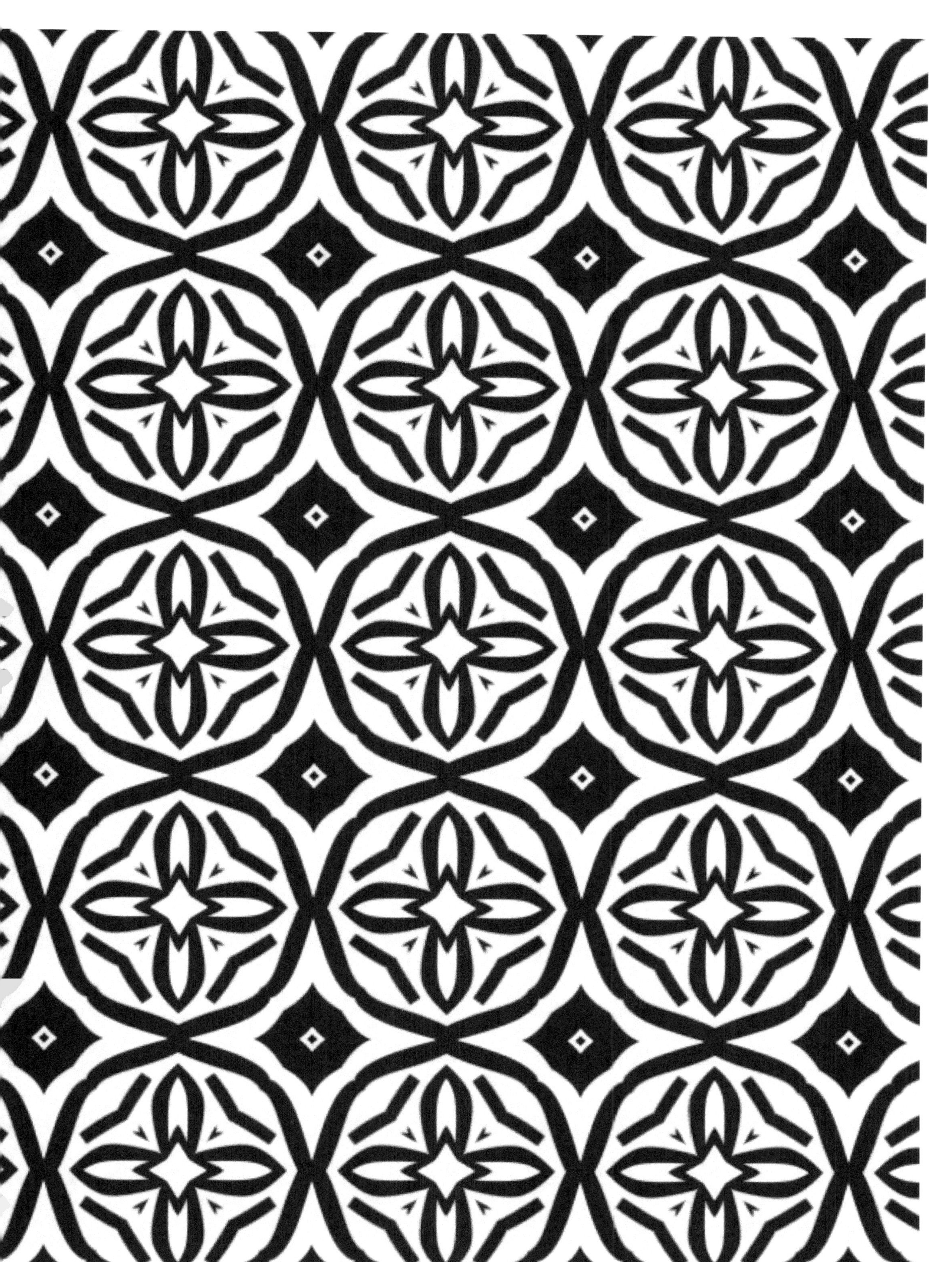

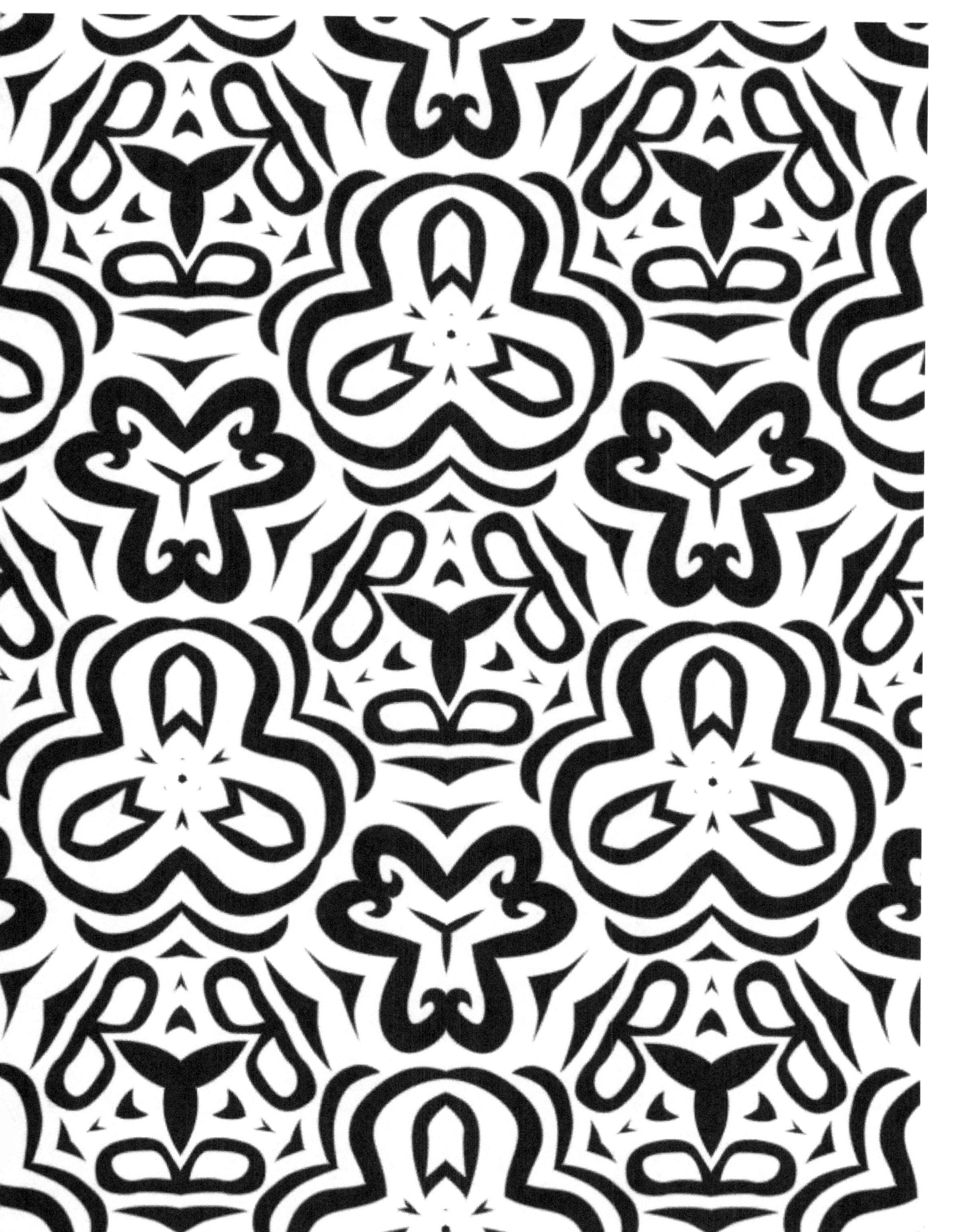

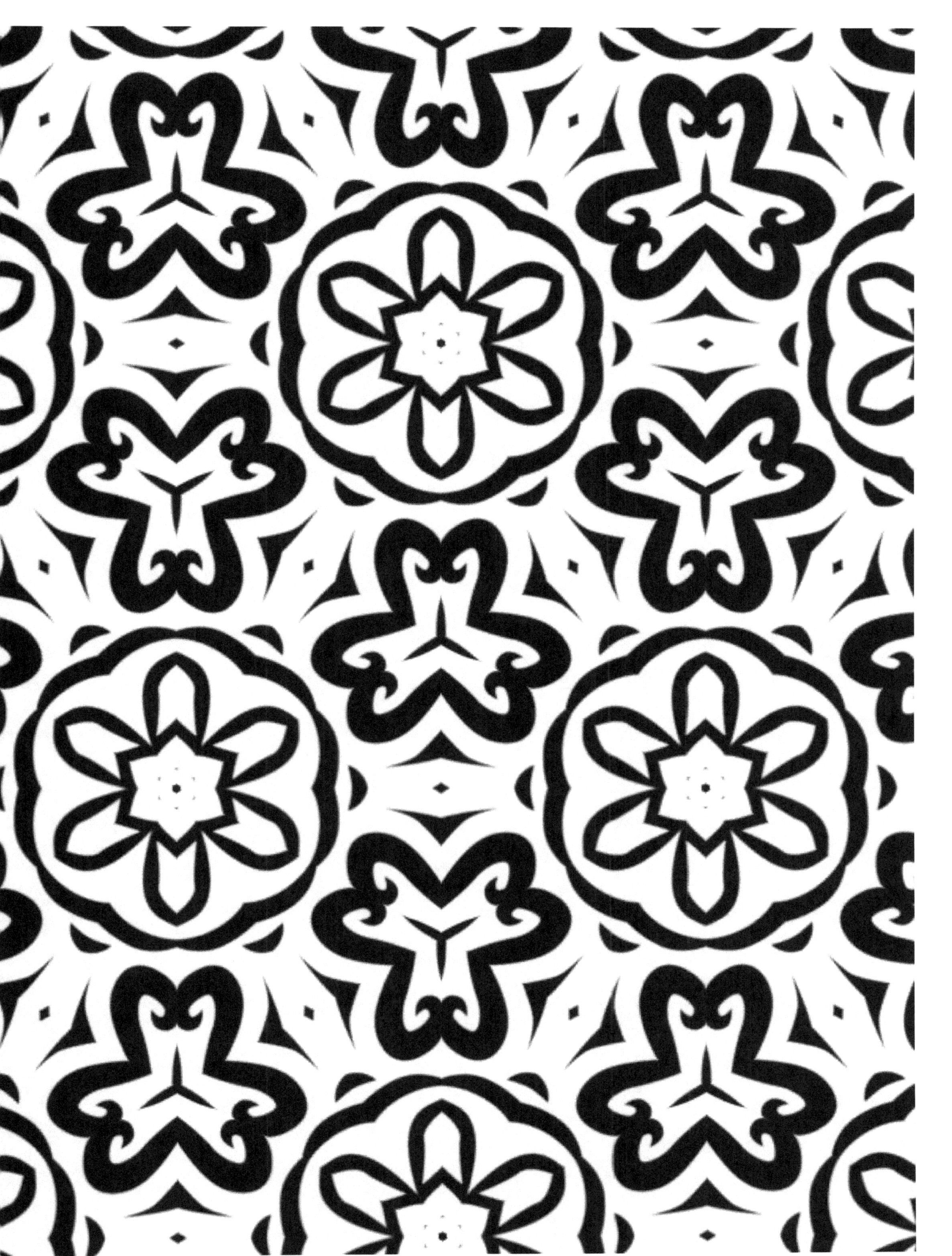

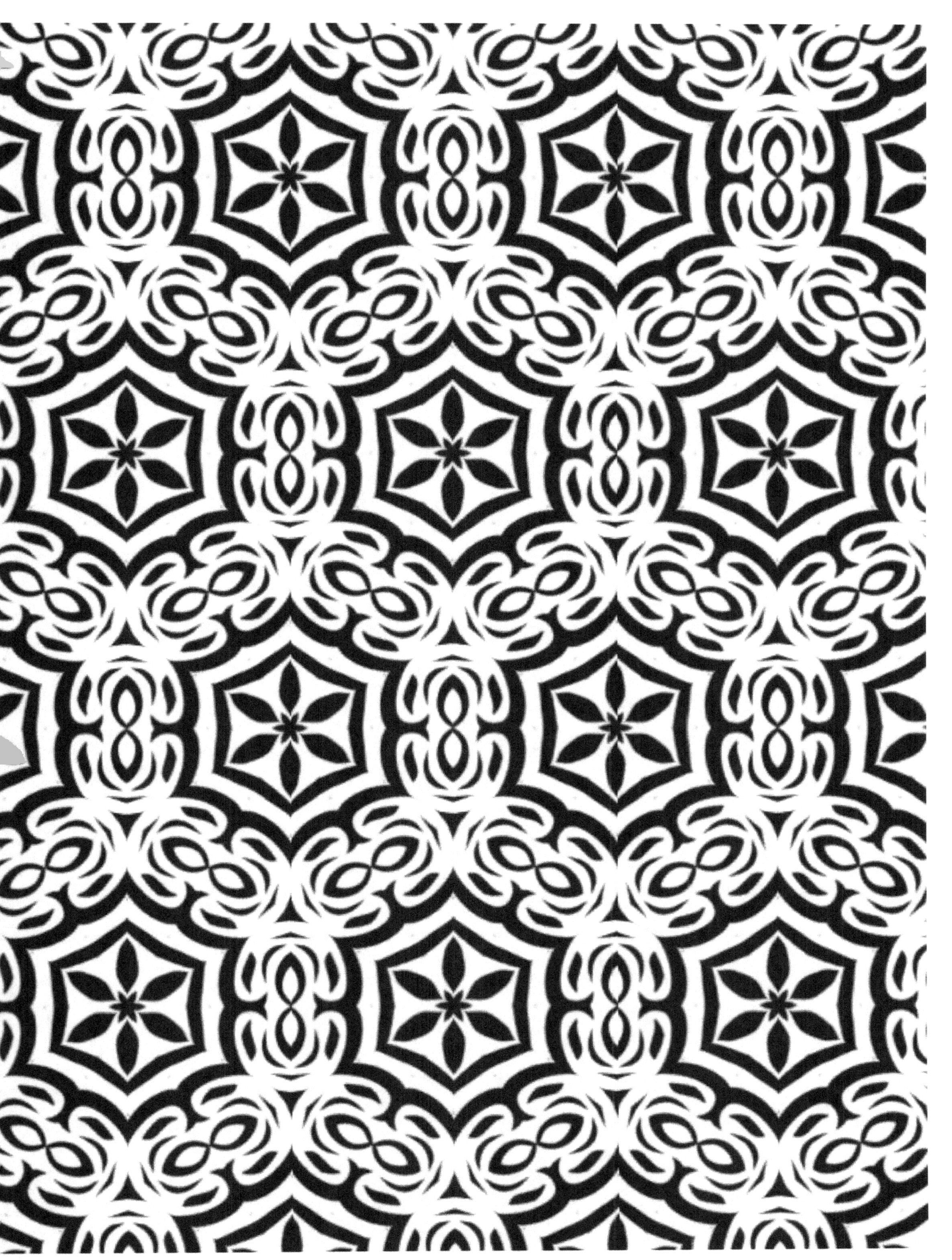

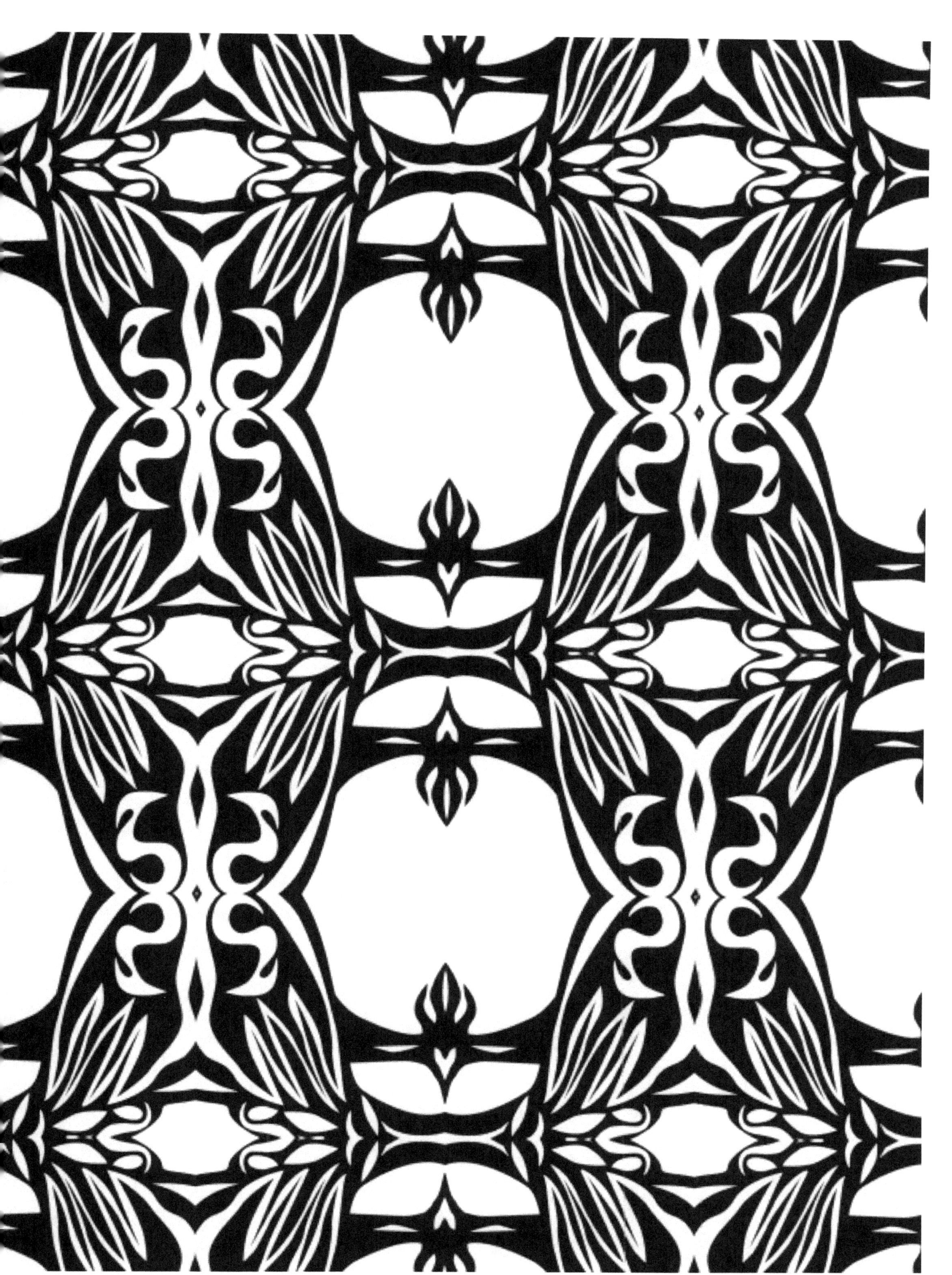

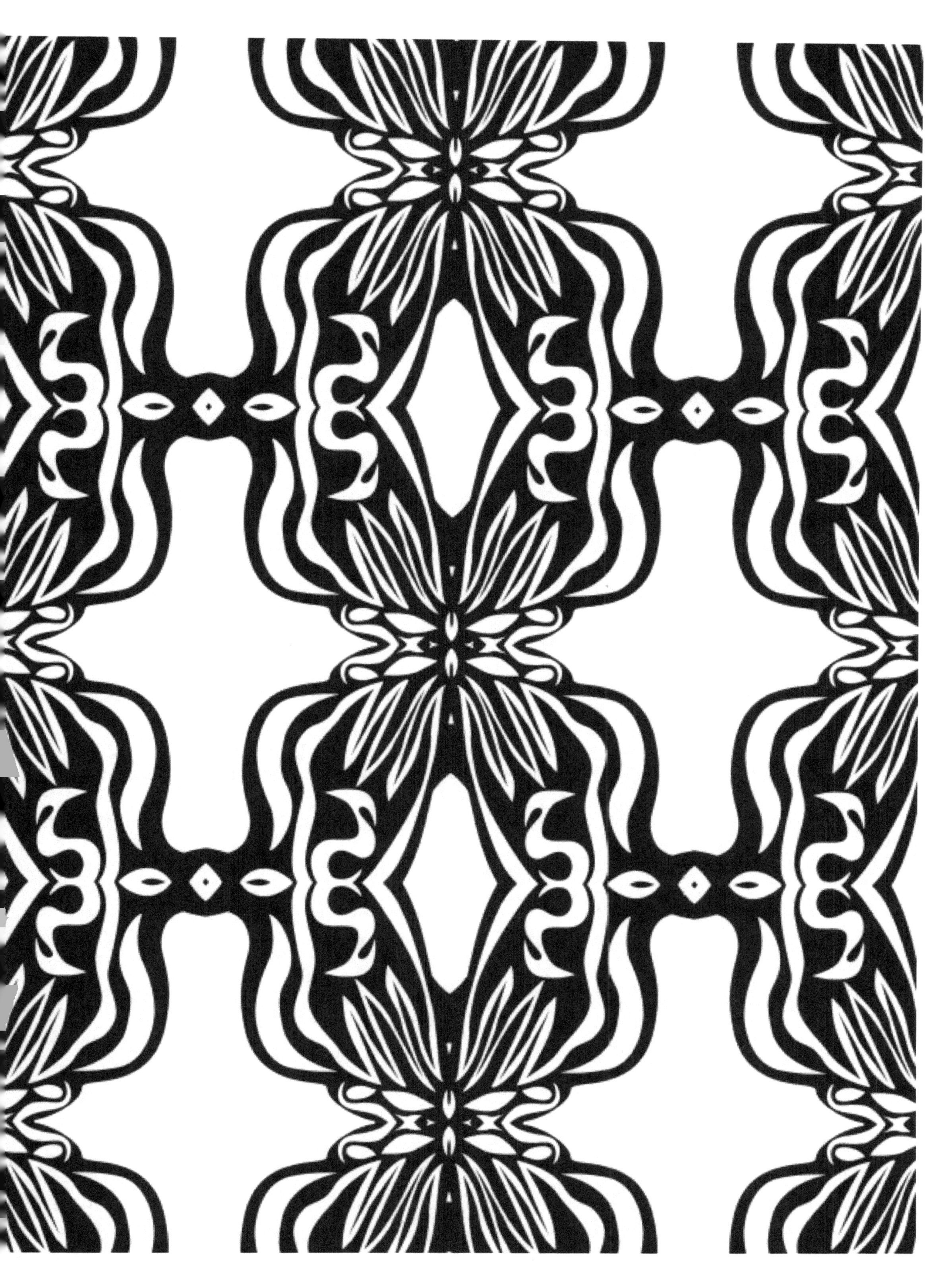

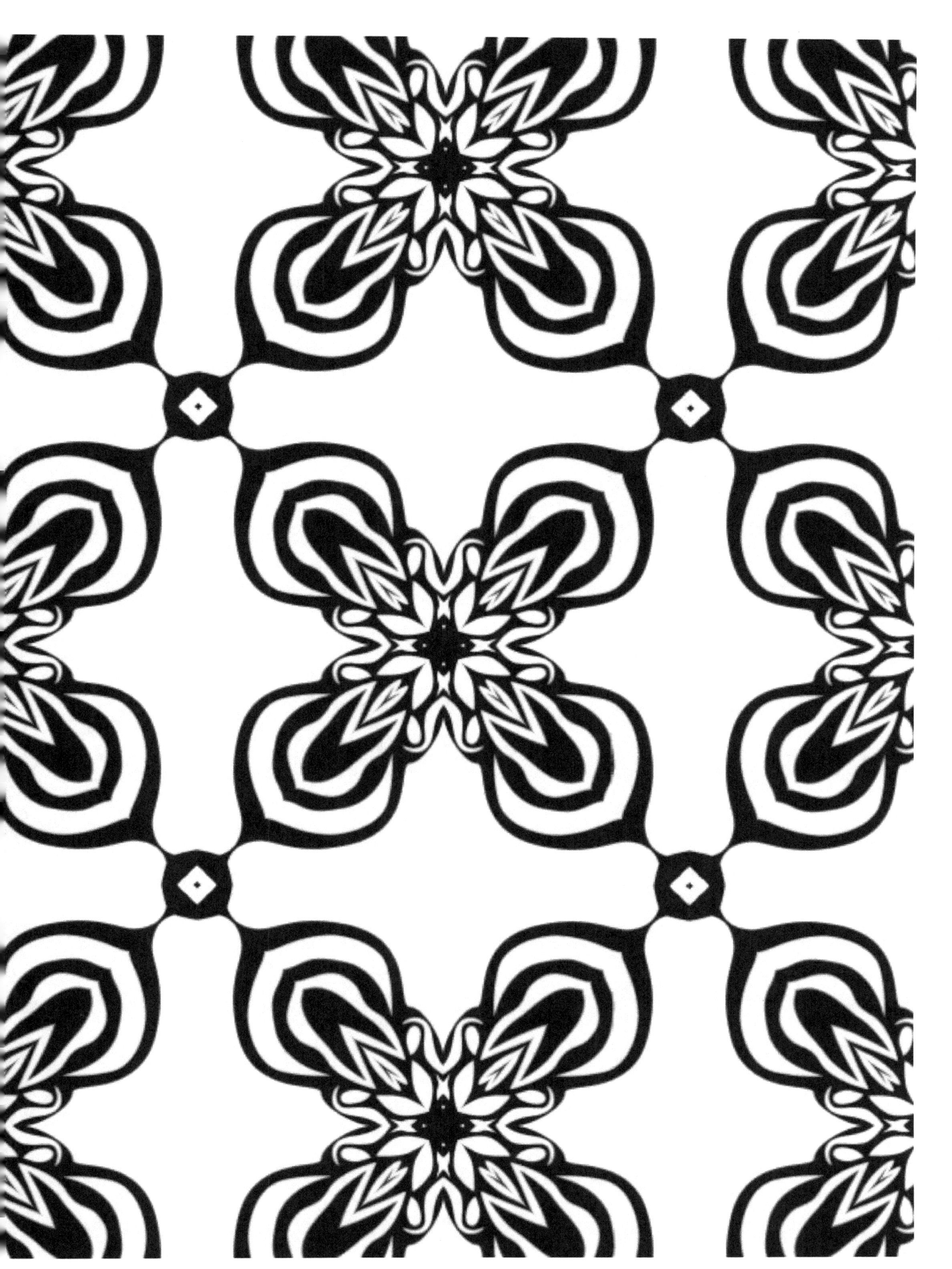

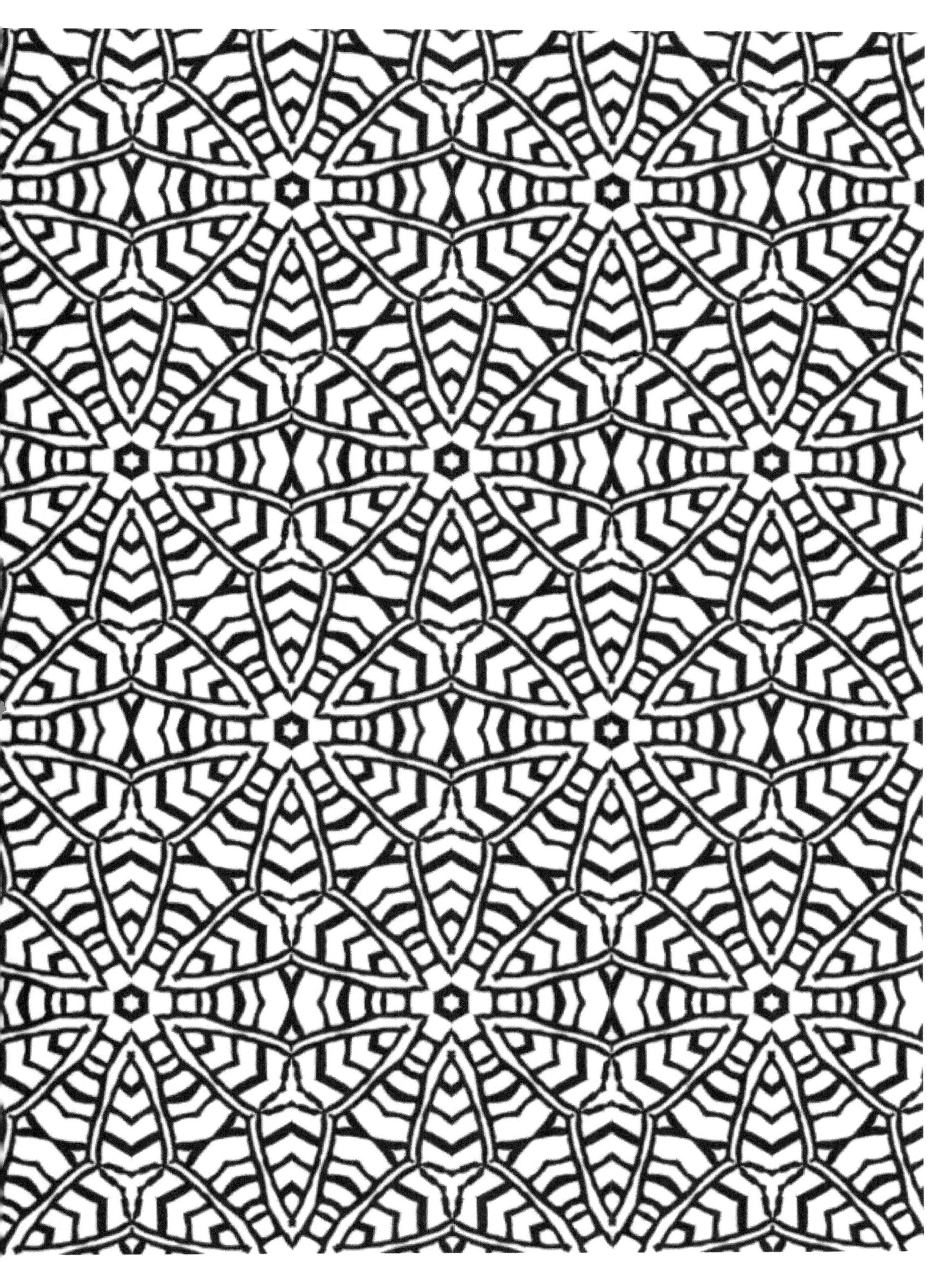

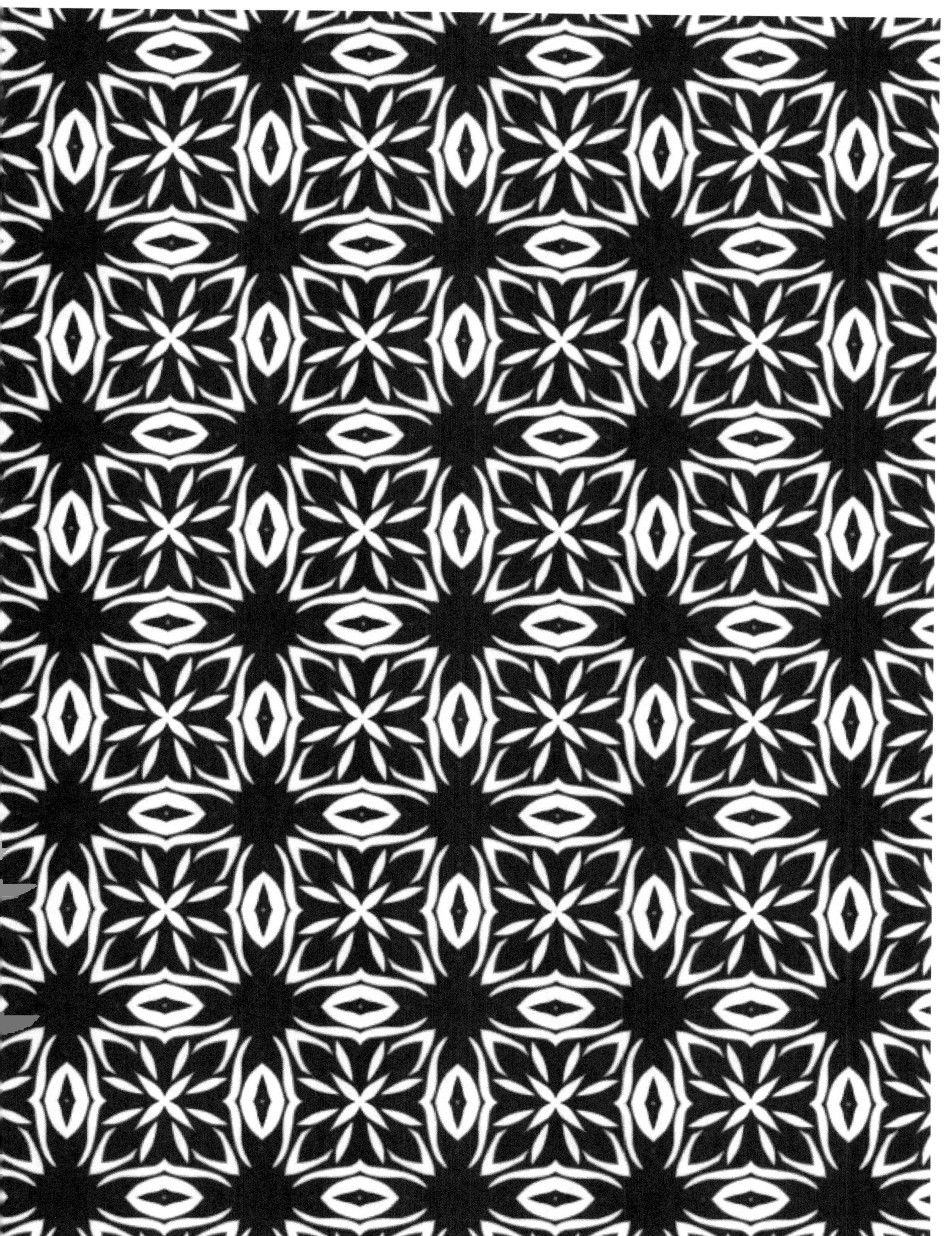

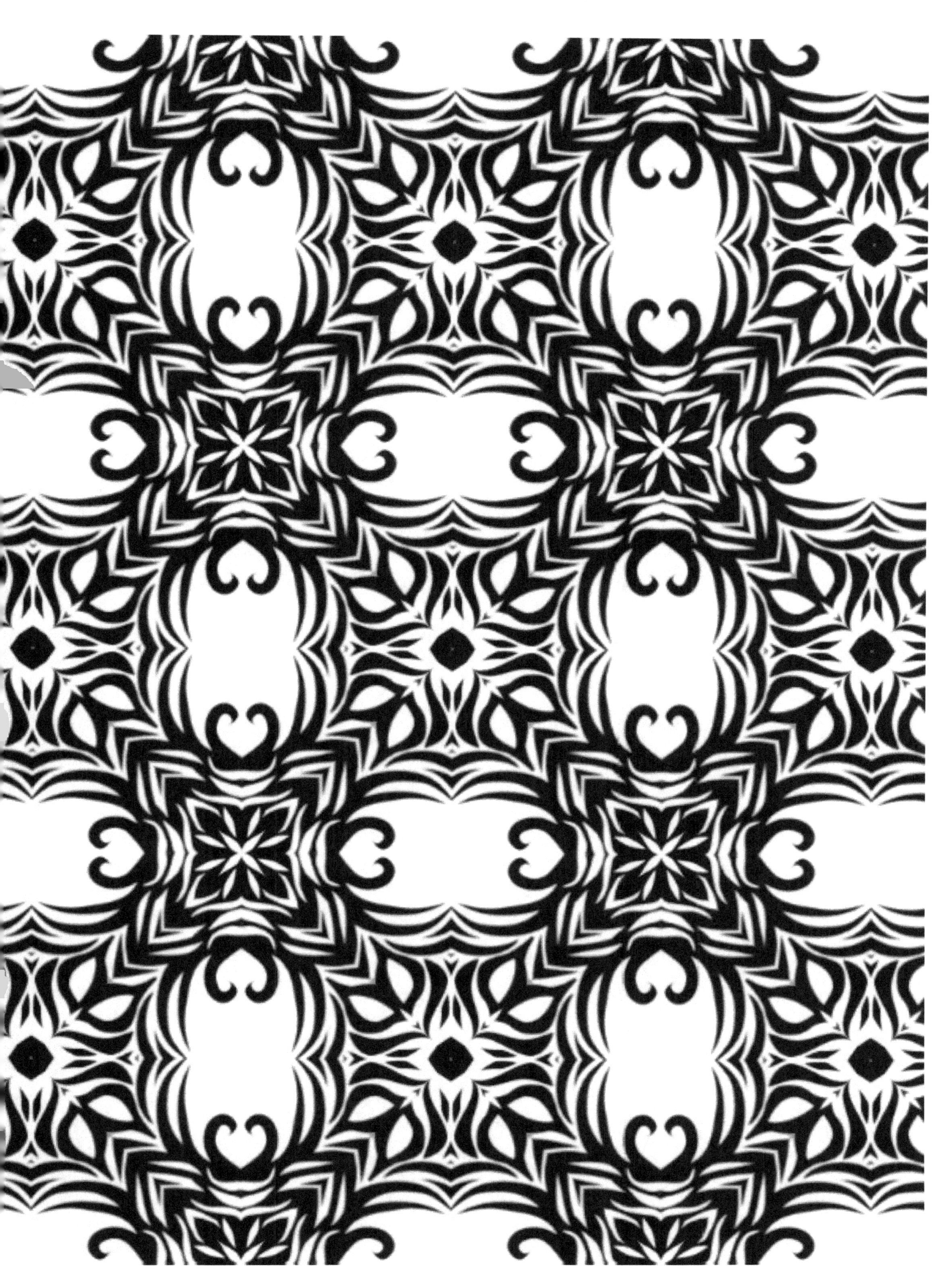

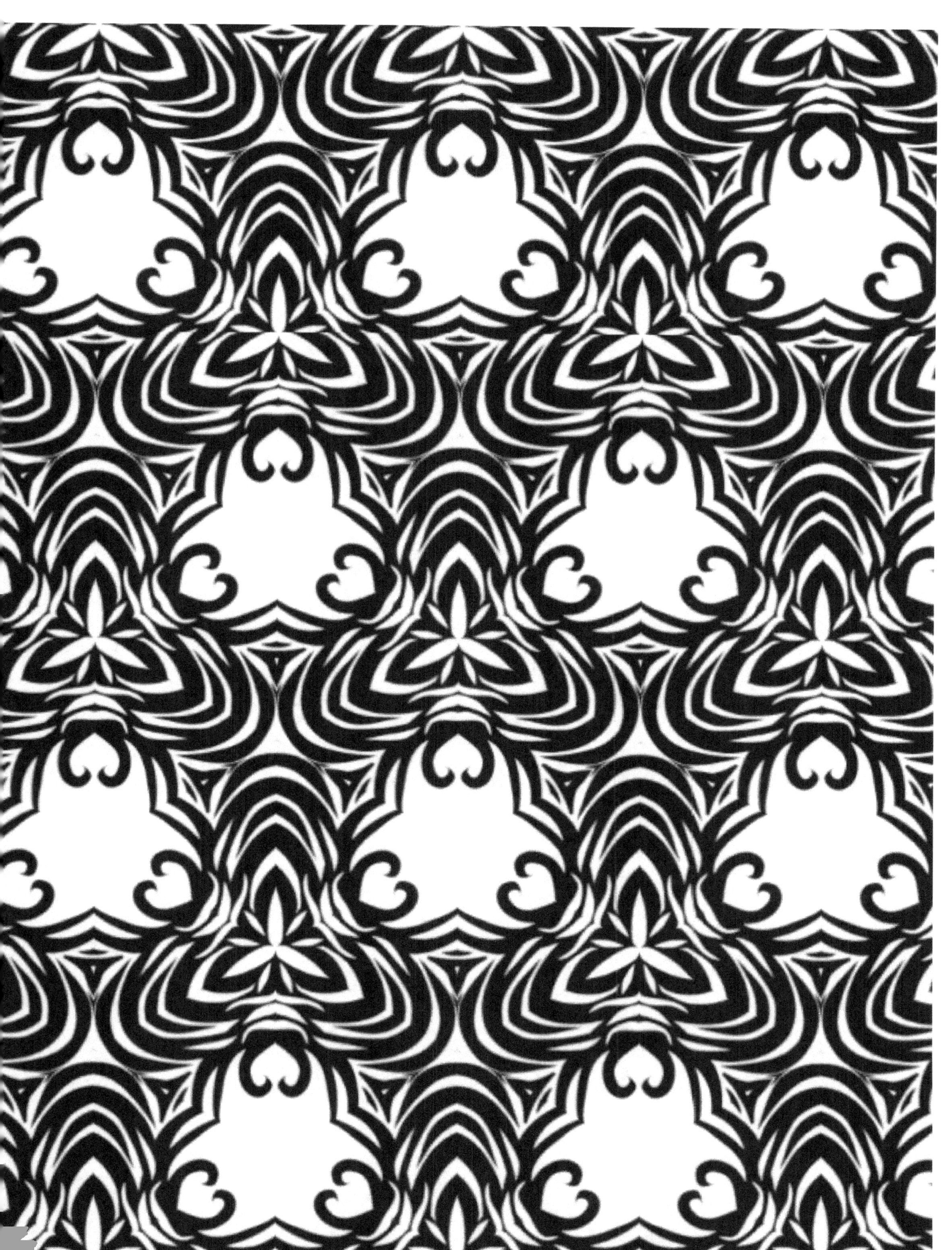

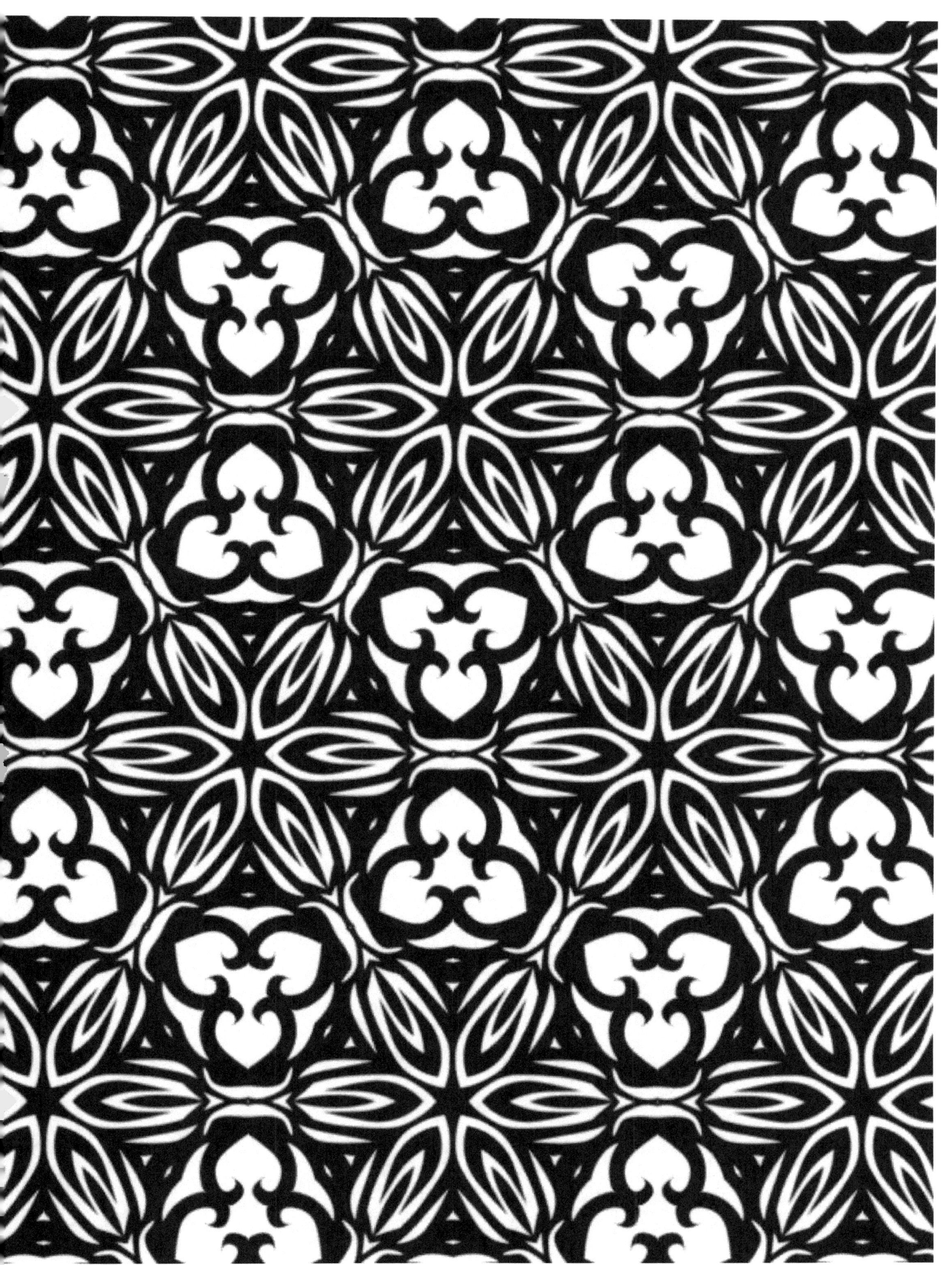

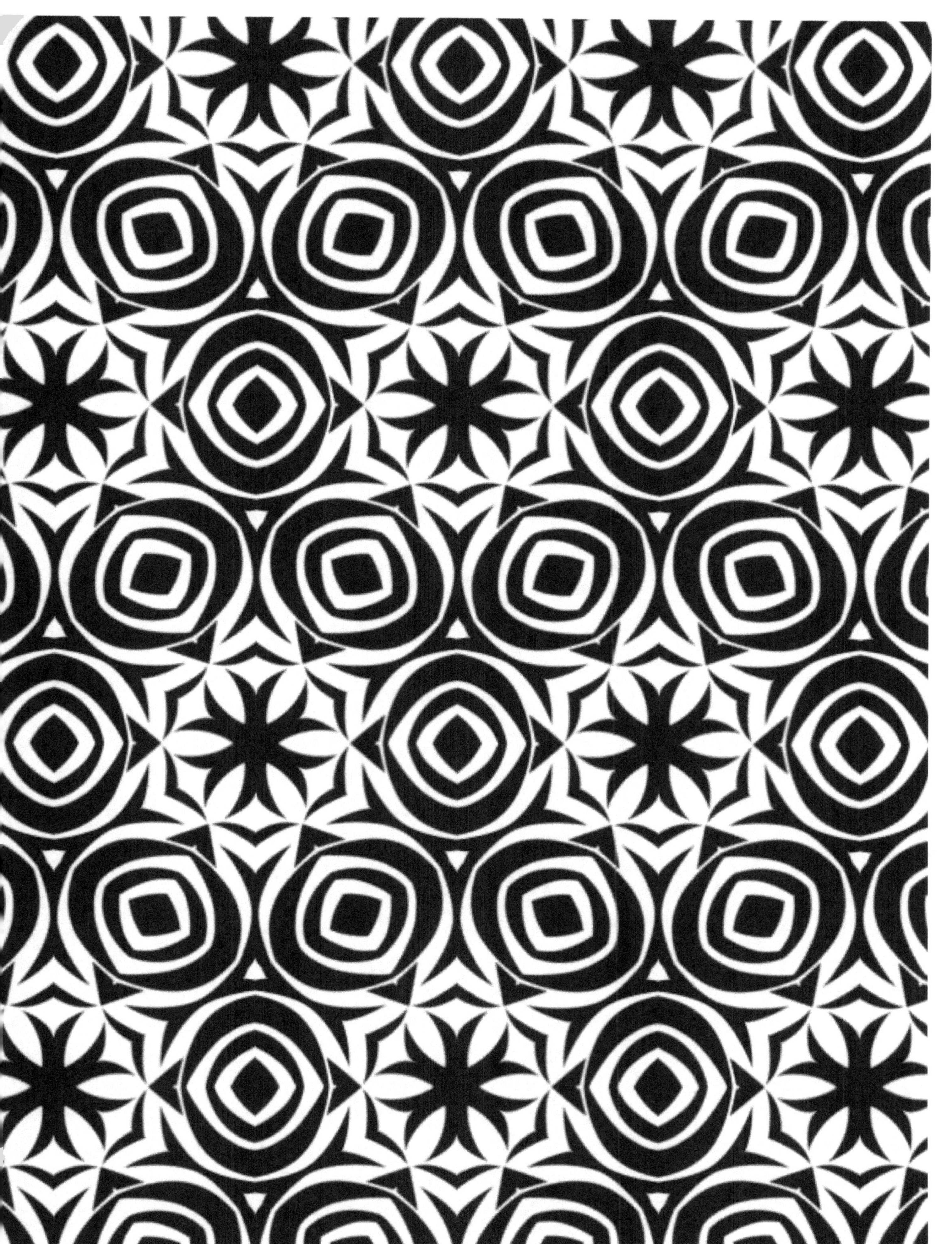

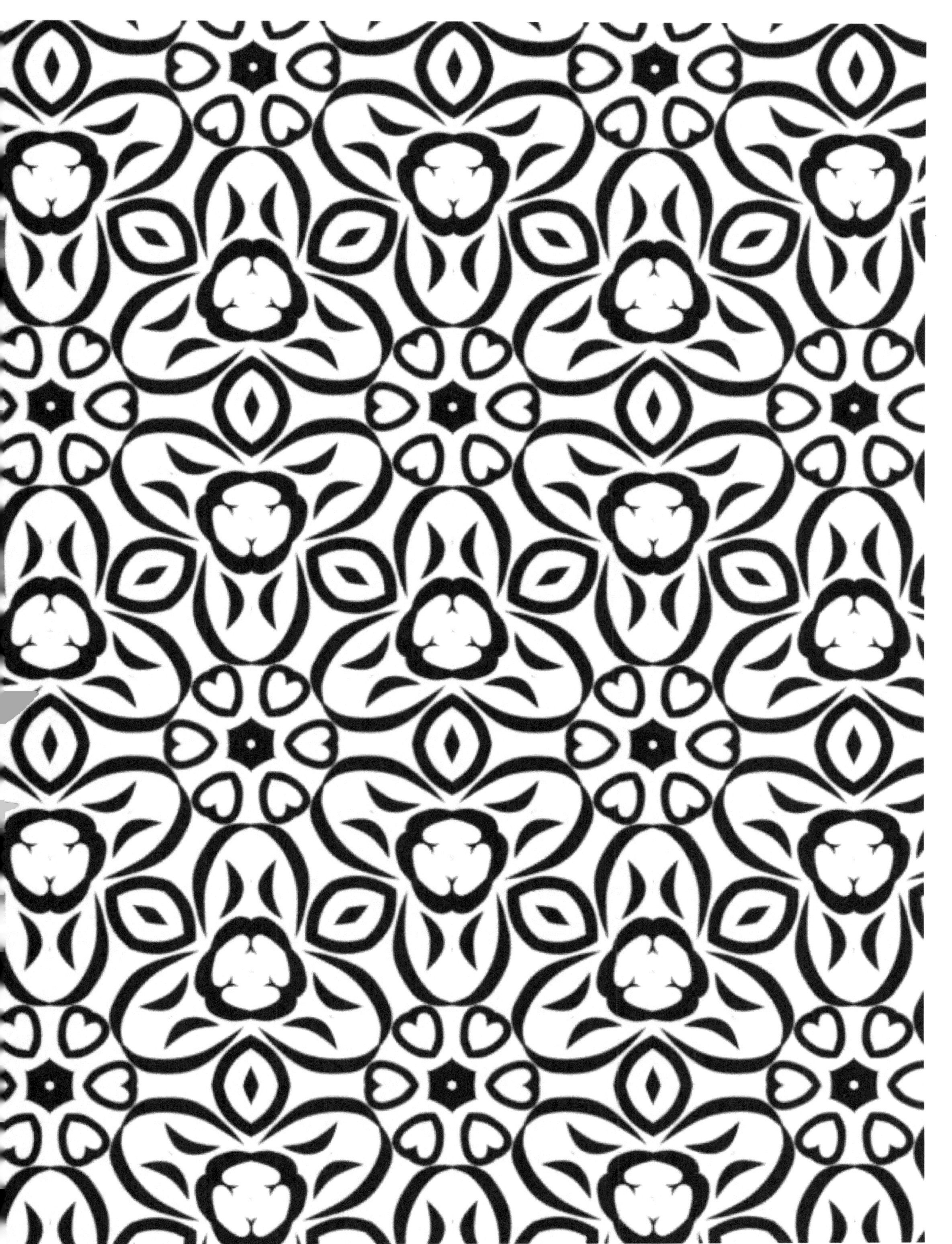

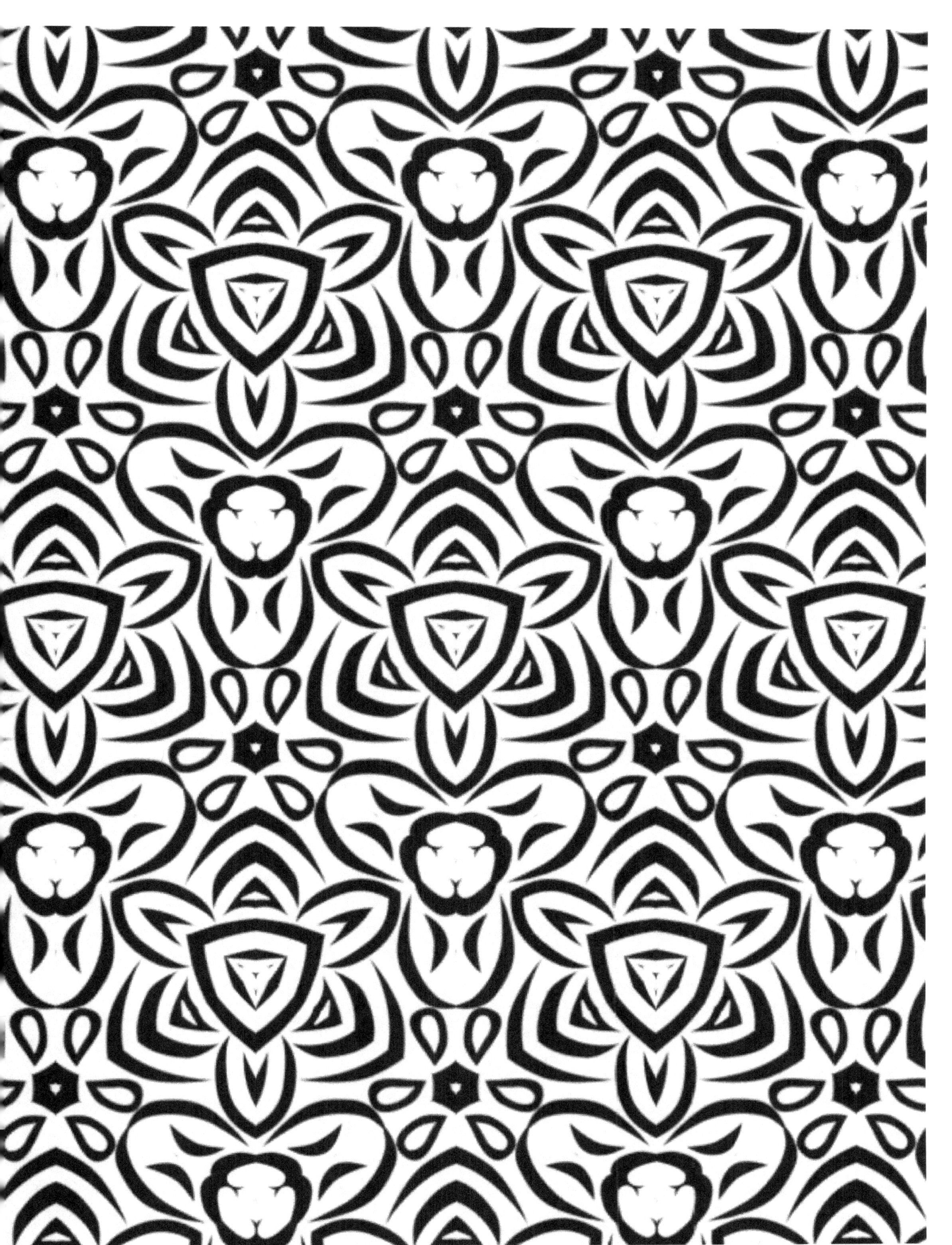

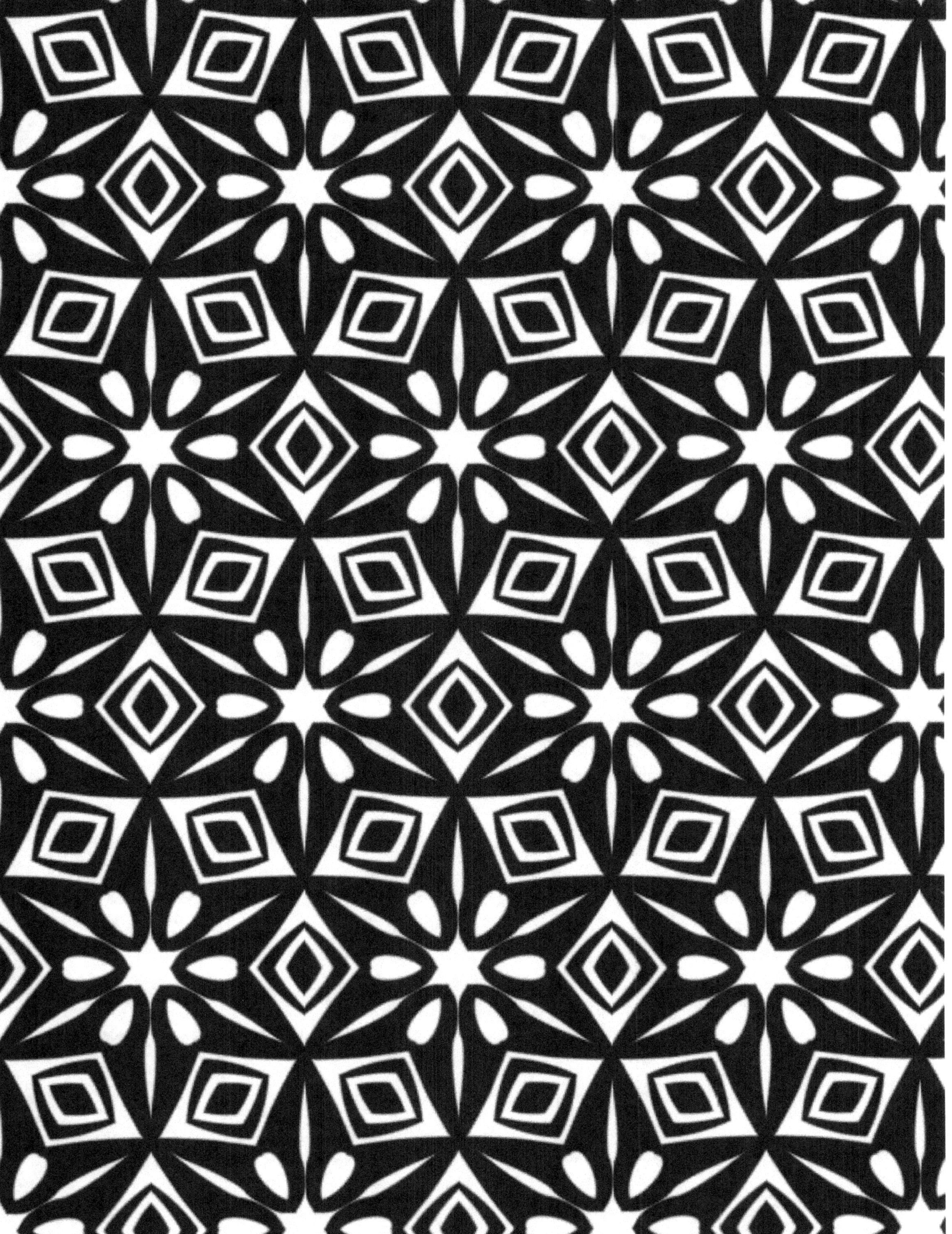

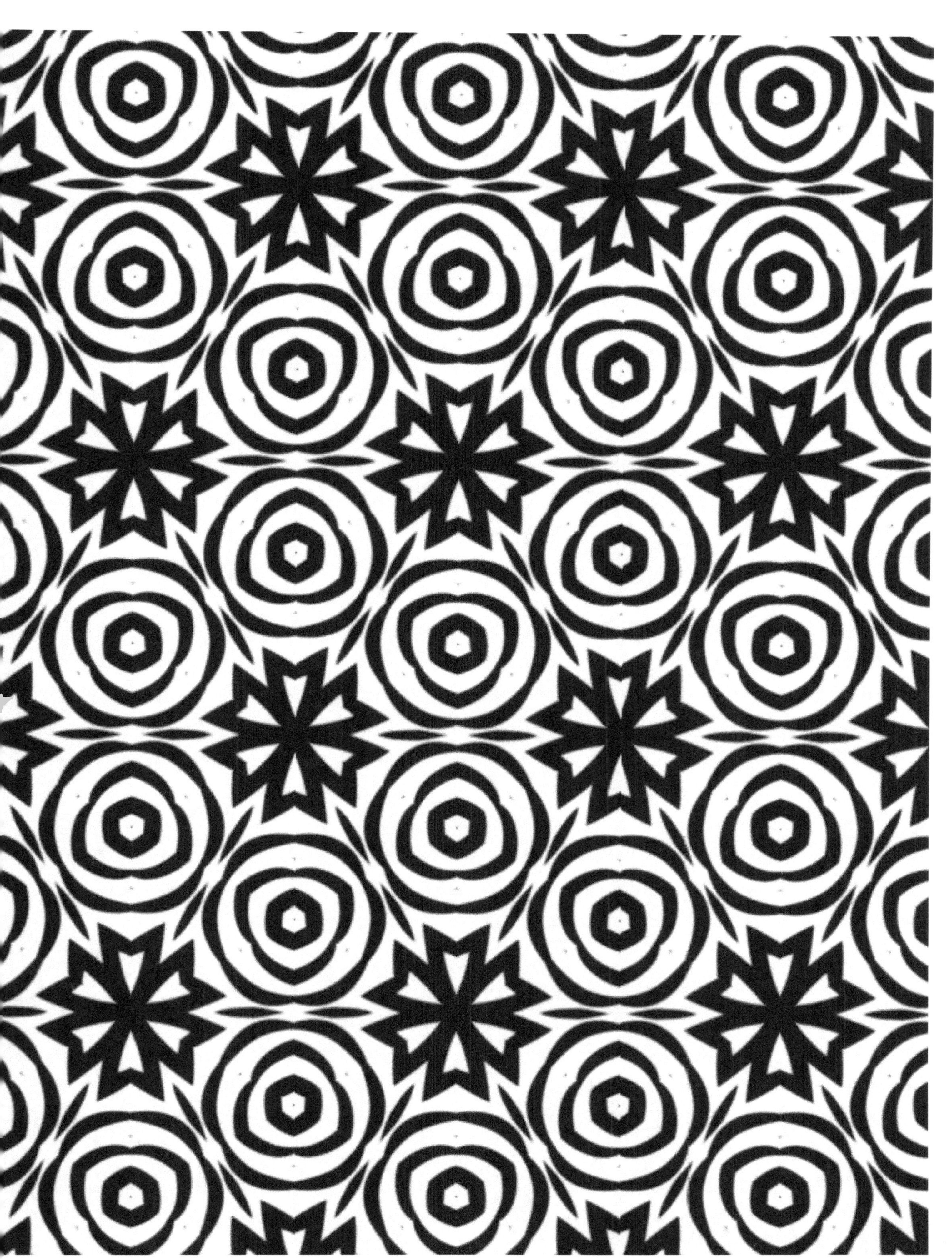